Quality Improvement and Implementation Science

Editors

MEGHAN B. LANE-FALL
LEE A. FLEISHER

ANESTHESIOLOGY CLINICS

www.anesthesiology.theclinics.com

Consulting Editor
LEE A. FLEISHER

March 2018 • Volume 36 • Number 1

ELSEVIER

1600 John F. Kennedy Boulevard • Suite 1800 • Philadelphia, Pennsylvania, 19103-2899

http://www.theclinics.com

ANESTHESIOLOGY CLINICS Volume 36, Number 1
March 2018 ISSN 1932-2275, ISBN-13: 978-0-323-58142-4

Editor: Colleen Dietzler
Developmental Editor: Kristen Helm

Photocopying

Single photocopies of single articles may be made for personal use as allowed by national copyright laws. Permission of the Publisher and payment of a fee is required for all other photocopying, including multiple or systematic copying, copying for advertising or promotional purposes, resale, and all forms of document delivery. Special rates are available for educational institutions that wish to make photocopies for non-profit educational classroom use. For information on how to seek permission visit www.elsevier.com/permissions or call: (+44) 1865 843830 (UK)/(+1) 215 239 3804 (USA).

Derivative Works

Subscribers may reproduce tables of contents or prepare lists of articles including abstracts for internal circulation within their institutions. Permission of the Publisher is required for resale or distribution outside the institution. Permission of the Publisher is required for all other derivative works, including compilations and translations (please consult www.elsevier.com/permissions).

Electronic Storage or Usage

Permission of the Publisher is required to store or use electronically any material contained in this periodical, including any article or part of an article (please consult www.elsevier.com/permissions). Except as outlined above, no part of this publication may be reproduced, stored in a retrieval system or transmitted in any form or by any means, electronic, mechanical, photocopying, recording or otherwise, without prior written permission of the Publisher.

Notice

No responsibility is assumed by the Publisher for any injury and/or damage to persons or property as a matter of products liability, negligence or otherwise, or from any use or operation of any methods, products, instructions or ideas contained in the material herein. Because of rapid advances in the medical sciences, in particular, independent verification of diagnoses and drug dosages should be made.

Although all advertising material is expected to conform to ethical (medical) standards, inclusion in this publication does not constitute a guarantee or endorsement of the quality or value of such product or of the claims made of it by its manufacturer.

Anesthesiology Clinics (ISSN 1932-2275) is published quarterly by Elsevier Inc., 360 Park Avenue South, New York, NY 10010-1710. Months of issue are March, June, September, and December. Periodicals postage paid at New York, NY and at additional mailing offices. Subscription prices are $100.00 per year (US student/resident), $346.00 per year (US individuals), $437.00 per year (Canadian individuals), $657.00 per year (US institutions), $830.00 per year (Canadian institutions), $225.00 per year (Canadian and foreign student/resident), $460.00 per year (foreign individuals), and $830.00 per year (foreign institutions). To receive student and resident rate, orders must be accompanied by name of affiliated institution, date of term, and the *signature* of program/residency coordinator on institutions letterhead. Orders will be billed at individual rate until proof of status is received. Foreign air speed delivery is included in all *Clinics'* subscription prices. All prices are subject to change without notice. POSTMASTER: Send address changes to *Anesthesiology Clinics,* Elsevier Health Sciences Division, Subscription Customer Service, 3251 Riverport Lane, Maryland Heights, MO 63043. Customer Service (orders, claims, online, change of address): Elsevier Health Sciences Division, Subscription Customer Service, 3251 Riverport Lane, Maryland Heights, MO 63043. **Tel:1-800-654-2452 (U.S. and Canada); 314-447-8871 (outside U.S. and Canada). Fax: 314-447-8029. E-mail: journalscustomerservice-usa@elsevier. com (for print support); journalsonlinesupport-usa@elsevier.com (for online support)**.

Reprints. For copies of 100 or more of articles in this publication, please contact the Commercial Reprints Department, Elsevier Inc., 360 Park Avenue South, New York, NY 10010-1710. Tel.: 212-633-3874; Fax: 212-633-3820; E-mail: reprints@elsevier.com.

Anesthesiology Clinics, is also published in Spanish by McGraw-Hill Inter-americana Editores S. A., P.O. Box 5-237, 06500 Mexico D. F., Mexico.

Anesthesiology Clinics, is covered in *MEDLINE/PubMed (Index Medicus), Current Contents/Clinical Medicine, Excerpta Medica, ISI/BIOMED*, and *Chemical Abstracts*.

Contributors

CONSULTING EDITOR

LEE A. FLEISHER, MD, FACC, FAHA
Robert D. Dripps Professor and Chair of Anesthesiology and Critical Care, Professor of Medicine, Perelman School of Medicine University of Pennsylvania, Philadelphia, Pennsylvania, USA

EDITORS

MEGHAN B. LANE-FALL, MD, MSHP
Assistant Professor of Anesthesiology and Critical Care, Co-Director, Penn Center for Perioperative Outcomes Research and Transformation, Perelman School of Medicine, Senior Fellow, Leonard Davis Institute of Health Economics, University of Pennsylvania, Philadelphia, Pennsylvania, USA

LEE A. FLEISHER, MD, FACC, FAHA
Robert D. Dripps Professor and Chair of Anesthesiology and Critical Care, Professor of Medicine, Perelman School of Medicine University of Pennsylvania, Philadelphia, Pennsylvania, USA

AUTHORS

AALOK V. AGARWALA, MD, MBA
Division Chief, General Surgery Anesthesia, Associate Director, Quality and Safety, Department of Anesthesia, Critical Care, and Pain Medicine, Massachusetts General Hospital, Instructor in Anesthesia, Harvard Medical School, Boston, Massachusetts, USA

ATILIO BARBEITO, MD, MPH
Co-Director, Quality Improvement, Assistant Professor, Department of Anesthesiology, Duke University Medical Center, Durham VA Health Care System, Durham, North Carolina, USA

SARAH BAUM, PhD
Postdoctoral Fellow, Institute for Learning and Brain Sciences, University of Washington, Seattle, Washington, USA

RINAD S. BEIDAS, PhD
Senior Fellow, Leonard Davis Institute of Health Economics, Assistant Professor of Psychiatry, Co-Director, Implementation Science Working Group, University of Pennsylvania, Philadelphia, Pennsylvania, USA

MELISSA BELLOMY, MD
Anesthesia Chief Resident, Department of Anesthesiology, Vanderbilt University Medical Center, Nashville, Tennessee, USA

ELIZABETH BLICKENSDERFER, PhD
Professor, Human Factors, Embry-Riddle Aeronautical University, Daytona Beach, Florida, USA

AMANDA BURDEN, MD
Associate Professor of Anesthesiology, Cooper Medical School of Rowan University, Camden, New Jersey, USA

KENDALL BURDICK, BS
Research Assistant, Neuroscience/Pre-Med Undergraduate, Vanderbilt University, Nashville, Tennessee, USA

CHRISTIE BURGER, PharmD
Clinical Pharmacist, Tennessee Valley Healthcare System, Nashville, Tennessee, USA

CRYSTAL WILEY CENÉ, MD, MPH
Associate Professor of Medicine, Division of General Internal Medicine, University of North Carolina at Chapel Hill School of Medicine, Chapel Hill, North Carolina, USA

ALEX CHERN, PhD
Medical Student, Vanderbilt University Medical Center, Nashville, Tennessee, USA

KRISTIN CHROUSER, MD
Assistant Professor, Department of Urology, University of Minnesota, Minneapolis, Minnesota, USA

BENJAMIN T. COBB, MD
Clinical Associate, Department of Anesthesiology and Critical Care, Perelman School of Medicine, Research Fellow, National Clinician Scholar Program, University of Pennsylvania, Philadelphia, Pennsylvania, USA

WILLIAM DANIEL, MD
Vice President and Chief Quality Officer, Office of the Executive Vice President for Health System Affairs, Professor of Internal Medicine (Cardiology) and Holder, William T. Solomon Professorship, Clinical Quality Improvement, The University of Texas Southwestern Medical Center, Dallas, Texas, USA

ELIZABETH M. ELLIOTT, MD
Assistant Professor, Department of Anesthesiology and Critical Care Medicine, Children's Hospital of Philadelphia, Perelman School of Medicine University of Pennsylvania, Philadelphia, Pennsylvania, USA

SCOTT A. FALK, MD
Associate Professor of Anesthesiology and Critical Care, Perelman School of Medicine University of Pennsylvania, Hospital of the University of Pennsylvania, Philadelphia, Pennsylvania, USA

YEHOSHUA GLEICHER, MSc, MD, FRCP
Lecturer, Anesthesiology, Mount Sinai Health Centre, University of Toronto, Toronto, Ontario, Canada

SARA N. GOLDHABER-FIEBERT, MD
Clinical Associate Professor, Department of Anesthesiology, Perioperative and Pain Medicine, Stanford University School of Medicine, Stanford, California, USA

PHILIP E. GREILICH, MD, FASE
Health System Quality Officer, Office of the Executive Vice President for Health System Affairs, S.T. "Buddy" Harris Chair Distinguished Chair, Cardiac Anesthesiology, Professor, Department of Anesthesiology and Pain Management, The University of Texas Southwestern Medical Center, Dallas, Texas, USA

KATHLEEN A. HARRIS, MD
Assistant Professor, Department of Anesthesiology and Critical Care Medicine, Children's Hospital of Philadelphia, Perelman School of Medicine University of Pennsylvania, Philadelphia, Pennsylvania, USA

JOSEPH R. KEEBLER, PhD
Assistant Professor, Human Factors, Embry-Riddle Aeronautical University, Daytona Beach, Florida, USA

MEGHAN B. LANE-FALL, MD, MSHP
Assistant Professor of Anesthesiology and Critical Care, Co-Director, Penn Center for Perioperative Outcomes Research and Transformation, Perelman School of Medicine, Senior Fellow, Leonard Davis Institute of Health Economics, University of Pennsylvania, Philadelphia, Pennsylvania, USA

ELIZABETH H. LAZZARA, PhD
Assistant Professor, Human Factors, Embry-Riddle Aeronautical University, Daytona Beach, Florida, USA

THOMAS D. LOOKE, PhD, MD
Anesthesiologist, Department of Anesthesiology, Florida Hospital Winter Park, Winter Park, Florida, USA; US Anesthesia Partners, Fort Lauderdal, Florida, USA; Florida Hospital, Orlando, Florida, USA

AMANDA LORINC, MD
Assistant Professor, Director, Pediatric Liver Transplant Anesthesiology, Division of Pediatric Anesthesiology, Monroe Carell Jr. Children's Hospital at Vanderbilt, Nashville, Tennessee, USA

ALISTAIR MacDONALD, MD
Staff Anesthesiologist, St. Patrick's University Hospital, Missoula, Montana, USA

CARL MACRAE, PhD
Visiting Senior Research Fellow, Department of Experimental Psychology, University of Oxford, Oxford, United Kingdom

IRENE McGHEE, MD, FRCP
Associate Professor, Anesthesiology, Sunnybrook Health Sciences Centre, University of Toronto, Toronto, Ontario, Canada

DOROTHEE MUELLER, MD
Assistant Professor, Department of Anesthesiology, Division of Critical Care Medicine, Vanderbilt University Medical Center, Nashville, Tennessee, USA

MARY ELEANOR PHELPS, MA, RN
Director of Nursing Quality Improvement, Office of the Associate Dean for Quality, Safety, and Outcomes Education, The University of Texas Southwestern Medical Center, Dallas, Texas, USA

ERIN WHITE PUKENAS, MD
Assistant Professor of Anesthesiology, Cooper Medical School of Rowan University, Camden, New Jersey, USA

LAURA E. SCHLEELEIN, MD
Assistant Professor, Department of Anesthesiology and Critical Care Medicine, Children's Hospital of Philadelphia, Perelman School of Medicine University of Pennsylvania, Philadelphia, Pennsylvania, USA

JOSEPH J. SCHLESINGER, MD
Assistant Professor, Department of Anesthesiology, Division of Critical Care Medicine, Vanderbilt University Medical Center, Nashville, Tennessee, USA; Assistant Professor of Electrical and Computer Engineering, McGill University, Montreal, Canada

ELIZABETH A. VALENTINE, MD
Assistant Professor of Anesthesiology and Critical Care, Perelman School of Medicine University of Pennsylvania, Hospital of the University of Pennsylvania, Philadelphia, Pennsylvania, USA

Contents

There is a 17-year gap between the initial publication of scientific evidence and its uptake into widespread practice in health care. The field of implementation science (IS) emerged in the 1990s as an answer to this "evidence-to-practice gap." In this article, the authors present an overview of implementation science, focusing on the application of IS principles to perioperative care. They describe opportunities for additional training and discuss strategies for funding and publishing IS work. The objective is to demonstrate how IS can improve perioperative patient care, while highlighting perioperative IS studies and identifying areas in need of additional investigation.

This article discusses some of the major theories of the science of human factors/ergonomics (HF/E) in relation to perioperative medicine, with a focus on safety and errors within these systems. The discussion begins with human limitations based in cognition, decision making, stress, and fatigue. Given these limitations, the importance of measuring human performance is discussed. Finally, using the HF/E perspective on safety, high-level recommendations are provided for increasing safety within the perioperative environment.

Quality improvement is at the heart of practice of anesthesiology. Objective data are critical for any quality improvement initiative; when possible, a combination of process, outcome, and balancing metrics should be evaluated to gauge the value of an intervention. Quality improvement is an ongoing process; iterative reevaluation of data is required to maintain interventions, ensure continued effectiveness, and continually improve.

Dashboards can facilitate rapid analysis of data and drive decision making. Large data sets can be useful to establish benchmarks and compare performance against other providers, practices, or institutions. Audit and feedback strategies are effective in facilitating positive change.

How can teams manage critical events more effectively? There are commonly gaps in performance during perioperative crises, and emergency manuals are recently available tools that can improve team performance under stress, via multiple mechanisms. This article examines how the principles of implementation science and quality improvement were applied by multiple teams in the development, testing, and systematic implementations of emergency manuals in perioperative care. The core principles of implementation have relevance for future patient safety innovations perioperatively and beyond, and the concepts of emergency manuals and interprofessional teamwork are applicable for diverse fields throughout health care.

Human error and system failures continue to play a substantial role in preventable errors that lead to adverse patient outcomes or death. Many of these deaths are not the result of inadequate medical knowledge and skill but occur because of problems involving communication and team management. Anesthesiologists pioneered the use of simulation for medical education in an effort to improve physician performance and patient safety. This article explores the use of simulation for performance improvement. Educational theories that underlie effective simulation programs are described as driving forces behind the advancement of simulation in performance improvement.

There are several benefits to clinical registries as an information repository tool, ultimately lending itself to the acquisition of new knowledge. Registries have the unique advantage of garnering much data quickly and are, therefore, especially helpful for niche populations or low-prevalence diseases. They can be used to inform on the ideal structure, process, or outcome involving an identified population. The data can be used in many ways, for example, as an observational tool to reveal associations or as a basis for framing future research studies or quality improvement projects.

Handovers around the time of surgery are common, yet complex and error prone. Interventions aimed at improving handovers have shown increased provider satisfaction and teamwork, improved efficiency, and improved communication and have been shown to reduce errors and improve clinical outcomes in some studies. Common recommendations in the literature include a standardized institutional process that allows flexibility among different units and settings, the completion of urgent tasks before information transfer, the presence of all members of the team for the duration of the handover, a structured conversation that uses a cognitive aid, and education in team skills and communication.

The concept of clinical workflow borrows from management and leadership principles outside of medicine. The only way to rethink clinical workflow is to understand the neuroscience principles that underlie attention and vigilance. With any implementation to improve practice, there are human factors that can promote or impede progress. Modulating the environment and working as a team to take care of patients is paramount. Clinicians must continually rethink clinical workflow, evaluate progress, and understand that other industries have something to offer. Then, novel approaches can be implemented to take the best care of patients.

Developing capacity to do improvement science starts with prioritizing quality improvement training in all health professions curricula so that a common knowledge base and understanding are created. Educational programs should include opportunities for colearning with patients, health professionals, and leaders. In this way, knowledge translation (also called implementation) is more effective and better coordinated when applied across organizations. Key factors that enable and drive behavior change are reviewed, as is the importance of influence and leadership. A comprehensive approach that accounts for these factors hardwires quality improvement into the health care systems and creates a culture that enables its ongoing development.

Diffusing innovation and best practices in healthcare are among the most challenging aspects of advancing patient safety and quality improvement. Recommendations from the Baldrige Foundation, Institute for Healthcare Improvement, and The Joint Commission provide guidance on the principles for successful diffusion. Perioperative leaders are encouraged to apply these principles to high priority areas such as handovers, enhanced recovery, and patient blood management. Completing a successful pilot project can be exciting; however, effective diffusion is essential to achieving meaningful and lasting impact on the service line and health system.

Quality Improvement and Implementation Science
ANESTHESIOLOGY CLINICS

THE CLINICS ARE AVAILABLE ONLINE!
Access your subscription at:
www.theclinics.com

Foreword

Improving Perioperative Care: What Are the Tools That Lead to Sustainable Change?

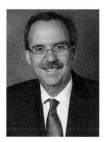

Lee A. Fleisher, MD, FACC, FAHA
Consulting Editor

The future of anesthesiology lies in our specialty's engagement in improving all aspects of perioperative care for the patient. While some have advocated the concept of the Perioperative Surgical Home, others have focused on perioperative medicine. The hallmark of either concept is change management and the ability to make the process culturally sensitive and that they "stick." Quality improvement is a formal approach to the analysis of performance and systematic efforts to improve it. Implementation Science is the study of methods to promote the integration of research findings and evidence into health care policy and practice. Together, they offer us the tools to provide high-quality care in a local environment.

This issue was edited by Meghan Lane-Fall, MD, MSHP and me. Dr Lane-Fall is currently Assistant Professor of Anesthesiology and Critical Care at the Perelman School of Medicine at the University of Pennsylvania. Her current research focuses on the impact of teamwork and communication on health care quality in the perioperative and critical care settings. Dr Lane-Fall has expertise in the use of mixed methods to answer health services research questions related to surgical care and critical illness. We have brought together a phenomenal group of authors to educate us on best current practices.

Lee A. Fleisher, MD, FACC, FAHA
Department of Anesthesiology and Critical Care
Perelman School of Medicine Health System
University of Pennsylvania
3400 Spruce Street, Dulles 680
Philadelphia, PA 19104, USA

E-mail address:
Lee.Fleisher@uphs.upenn.edu

Anesthesiology Clin 36 (2018) xi
https://doi.org/10.1016/j.anclin.2017.12.002
1932-2275/18/© 2017 Published by Elsevier Inc.

anesthesiology.theclinics.com

Preface

Quality Improvement and Implementation Science: Different Fields with Aligned Goals

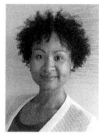 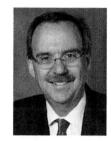

Meghan B. Lane-Fall, MD, MSHP   Lee A. Fleisher, MD, FACC, FAHA
Editors

One hundred years ago, Massachusetts surgeon Ernest Codman advocated the unpopular idea that physicians and hospitals should track patient outcomes to determine the effectiveness of the care rendered to these patients. This heretical concept caused friction with his contemporaries and administrators at the Massachusetts General Hospital, from which he resigned to start a private hospital where he could practice his End Result System that tracked patients and outcomes.[1,2]

Now, Codman's idea is accepted dogma. We recognize that patients' outcomes often fall short of our collective expectations. One important reason for this failure is that scientific evidence about patient care (including diagnosis and management) is unevenly and inconsistently applied. This phenomenon is known as the evidence-to-practice performance gap.

The evidence-practice performance gap is a natural target for health care improvement efforts. In this issue of *Anesthesiology Clinics*, we present articles addressing two distinct but complementary approaches to narrowing the performance gap: quality improvement (QI) and implementation science (IS).

QI and IS are part of a spectrum of approaches aimed at improving care quality to improve health outcomes. Although QI and IS share some assumptions and techniques (**Table 1**), an important difference is the focus on creating timely local change (QI) versus creating more explicitly theory-based generalizable knowledge that necessarily proceeds more slowly (IS).

Our detailed treatment of perioperative QI and IS starts with an explanation of how the relatively new field of IS can be leveraged to improve perioperative care (Lane-Fall and colleagues). Next, we explore the application of human factors/ergonomics to perioperative performance improvement (Keebler and colleagues), which is relevant

Anesthesiology Clin 36 (2018) xiii–xv
https://doi.org/10.1016/j.anclin.2017.12.001
1932-2275/18/© 2017 Published by Elsevier Inc.

Table 1
Similarities and differences between quality improvement operations, quality improvement science, and implementation science

	Quality Improvement Operations	Quality Improvement Science	Implementation Science
Assumptions	Evidence-based practices, benchmarks, guidelines exist, -or- there is variability in care or outcomes	Evidence-based practices, benchmarks, guidelines exist, -or- there is variability in care or outcomes	Evidence-based practices, benchmarks, or guidelines exist
Time focus	Initial focus on improvement in the *short term*, then focus on *sustainability* over time	Initial focus on improvement in the *short to medium term* (scientific rigor justifies taking more time), then focus on *sustainability* over time	Initial focus on improvement in the *medium to long term* (scientific rigor justifies taking more time), then focus on *sustainability* over time
Generalizability goal	Focused on *local practice*	Interested in applicability to *multiple settings*; characterization of context is essential	Applicability to *multiple settings* is essential, as is characterization of context
Use of explicit theoretical models	Not very important	Somewhat important	Extremely important
Common tools	Stakeholder analysis, rapid, small-scale tests of change, run and control charts, root and apparent cause analyses, process maps, flow charts; focused on *effectiveness outcomes*	Hypothesis-generating studies (often qualitative); prospective experimental and quasi-experimental studies focused on *effectiveness outcomes* (qualitative/quantitative/mixed methods)	Hypothesis-generating studies (often qualitative); prospective experimental and quasi-experimental studies focused on *implementation outcomes* (qualitative/quantitative/mixed methods)
Related disciplines	Leadership, change management Human factors/ergonomics	Human factors/ergonomics Management science	Behavior change theory Management science

to both QI and IS. Valentine and colleagues follow with a discussion of how to use data to drive QI. We then present strategies to improve performance: the use of crisis checklists (Goldhaber-Fiebert and Macrae) and simulation (Pukenas and Burden) as well as one tool to collect data for improvement efforts: patient registries (Schleelein and colleagues). We present cases for improvement work, including handoffs (Barbeito and colleagues) and an approach to reengineering clinical work (Schlesinger and colleagues), both of which employ strategies discussed in earlier articles. Finally, we conclude with an eye to the future, discussing how to build capacity to do improvement work (McGhee and colleagues) and spreading and scaling change to the health system level (Greilich and colleagues).

We hope that you find this collection to be interesting, thought-provoking, and useful. We genuinely appreciate the opportunity to offer guidance to perioperative clinicians and researchers interested in realizing the promise of evidence-based practice and optimal health care.

Meghan B. Lane-Fall, MD, MSHP
Department of Anesthesiology and Critical Care
Perelman School of Medicine
3400 Spruce Street, Dulles 680
Philadelphia, PA 19104, USA

Lee A. Fleisher, MD, FACC, FAHA
Department of Anesthesiology and Critical Care
Perelman School of Medicine Health System
University of Pennsylvania
3400 Spruce Street, Dulles 680
Philadelphia, PA 19104, USA

E-mail addresses:
Meghan.LaneFall@uphs.upenn.edu (M.B. Lane-Fall)
Lee.Fleisher@uphs.upenn.edu (L.A. Fleisher)

REFERENCES

1. Howell J, Ayanian J. Ernest Codman and the end result system: a pioneer of health outcomes revisited. J Health Serv Res Policy 2016;21(4):279–81.
2. Neuhauser D. Ernest Amory Codman MD. Qual Saf Health Care 2002;11(1):104–5.

Implementation Science in Perioperative Care

Meghan B. Lane-Fall, MD, MSHP[a,b,c,]*, Benjamin T. Cobb, MD[c,d],
Crystal Wiley Cené, MD, MPH[e], Rinad S. Beidas, PhD[b,f]

KEYWORDS

- Implementation science • Evidence-based practice • Evidence-practice gap
- Perioperative research

KEY POINTS

- The field of implementation science (IS) aims to routinize the use of evidence-based practice, narrowing the gap between evidence and real-world practice. The goal of IS is to produce generalizable knowledge to promote health through the uptake, and effective use of evidence-based practices.
- IS relies on the presence of interventions that have been studied and that have proven efficacy and effectiveness (ie, evidence-based practices).
- The use of the theories and frameworks helps guide the selection of implementation outcomes and strategies, and is essential in IS research.
- Hybrid effectiveness-implementation trials are one strategy to apply IS principles to the study of interventions with limited evidence of efficacy.
- Multiple perioperative care interventions have shown both evidence of improvements in patient outcomes and incomplete uptake and adherence (ie, an evidence-practice gap).

INTRODUCTION

There is a 17-year gap between the initial publication of scientific evidence and its uptake into widespread practice in health care.[1] This gap translates into lives lost, as well as potential waste of health care resources and unnecessary expense. The field of

Disclosure Statement: The authors have no financial relationships to disclose.
[a] Penn Center for Perioperative Outcomes Research and Transformation, Perelman School of Medicine, University of Pennsylvania, 423 Guardian Drive, 333 Blockley Hall, Philadelphia, PA 19104, USA; [b] Leonard Davis Institute of Health Economics, University of Pennsylvania, Colonial Penn Center, 3641 Locust Walk Philadelphia, PA 19104-6218; [c] Department of Anesthesiology and Critical Care, Perelman School of Medicine, University of Pennsylvania, 3400 Spruce Street, 680 Dulles (Anesthesia), Philadelphia, PA 19104, USA; [d] National Clinician Scholar Program, University of Pennsylvania, 423 Guardian Drive, 1310 Blockley Hall, Philadelphia, PA 19104, USA; [e] Division of General Internal Medicine, School of Medicine, University of North Carolina at Chapel Hill, 101 Manning Drive #1050, Chapel Hill, NC 27514, USA; [f] Implementation Science Working Group, University of Pennsylvania, 3535 Market Street, Suite 3015, Philadelphia, PA 19104, USA
* Corresponding author. 3400 Spruce Street, 680 Dulles (Anesthesia), Philadelphia, PA 19104.
E-mail address: LaneMe@upenn.edu

Anesthesiology Clin 36 (2018) 1–15
https://doi.org/10.1016/j.anclin.2017.10.004
1932-2275/18/© 2017 Elsevier Inc. All rights reserved.

implementation science (IS) emerged in the 1990s as an answer to this what has been termed an "evidence-to-practice gap."[2] The field of IS emerged as a way to systematically study the process of translating evidence into practice.

In this article, we present an overview of implementation science, focusing on the application of IS principles to perioperative care. We also describe opportunities for additional training and discuss strategies for funding and publishing IS work. The objective of this discussion, much like other discipline-specific overviews of IS,[3-5] is to demonstrate the potential value of IS approaches in one area: perioperative care. In so doing, we hope to demonstrate how IS can improve perioperative patient care, while highlighting perioperative IS studies and identifying areas in need of additional investigation.

WHAT IS IMPLEMENTATION SCIENCE?

In the inaugural issue of the flagship journal for the field, *Implementation Science*, Eccles and Mittman[6] offer the following definition of IS: "the scientific study of methods to promote the systematic uptake of research findings and other evidence-based practices into routine practice, and, hence, to improve the quality and effectiveness of health services and care." More recently, experts in IS have recommended that it include the concept of "de-implementation," or the discontinuation of practices known not to be effective.[7] Implementation is part of the spectrum of dissemination and implementation described by Rogers.[8] For the purposes of this discussion, we use the term "implementation science"; another term for the same area of study is "knowledge translation," primarily used in Canada.[9]

IS is complementary to, but distinct from, research focused on clinical efficacy and effectiveness. Studies of intervention efficacy (the degree to which an intervention works in an idealized research setting) and effectiveness (the degree to which an intervention works in the "real world") address the question: *"Does this intervention achieve the expected change(s) in health outcomes?"* In contrast, studies of implementation address questions such as *"Is the intervention being used?" "Are the procedures used to deliver the intervention being followed?"* and *"Can one particular strategy increase use of evidence-based practice compared with another strategy?"* These different questions make clear that effectiveness outcomes and implementation outcomes *are not the same*. Proctor and colleagues[10] published a model explaining the relationship between implementation outcomes, process outcomes, and patient outcomes. In the Proctor model, implementation outcomes influence process ("service") outcomes, which in turn influence patient ("client") outcomes. The National Academy of Medicine (formerly the Institute of Medicine) envisions IS as a key component of learning health care systems designed to iteratively develop innovations to deliver high-quality patient-centered care and to evaluate the effectiveness of this care.[11] Indeed, IS is central to addressing the "quality chasm" identified by the Institute of Medicine in 2001.[12]

HOW MIGHT IMPLEMENTATION SCIENCE ADVANCE OUR UNDERSTANDING OF PERIOPERATIVE CARE?

Implementation science is an interdisciplinary field broadly relevant to health and health care, and has been used in settings as distinct as mental, community, and public health.[13] In contrast, there are fewer IS studies relating to perioperative care. In this section, we discuss the potential for IS to facilitate the uptake and effective use of evidence-based perioperative interventions. We then highlight several perioperative studies using implementation science principles. For the purposes of this discussion, "perioperative care" includes care rendered by anesthesia and surgical teams, such as the preoperative assessment clinic, operating theater, postanesthesia care unit, intensive care unit, obstetrics ward, and pain clinic.

Potential for Implementation Research to Improve Perioperative Care

There are several important evidence-based practices that relate to perioperative care. IS has the potential to improve patient outcomes by deepening our understanding of the factors influencing adherence to evidence-based practices aimed at improving value and safety. Two examples of these evidence-based practices are enhanced recovery after surgery (ERAS) and the Safe Surgery Saves Lives Surgical Safety Checklist (SSC).

ERAS builds on the principles of fast-track surgery,[14] amounting to a multimodal perioperative care program designed to reduce recovery time, length of hospital admission, and most importantly, surgical complications. ERAS pathways include patient-engaged preoperative interventions (eg, carbohydrate-rich oral supplementation until 3 hours before surgery, no premedication), anesthesia-driven intraoperative interventions (eg, fluid restriction, multimodal analgesia, hypothermia prevention), and nursing-driven postoperative interventions (eg, early mobilization, limiting opioids, early detection and prevention of nausea and vomiting). By integrating these actions into perioperative care in the early 2000s, Kehlet and Mogensen[15] reported a 4.5-fold reduction in hospital admission time for colorectal surgery patients. Since then, meta-analyses of ERAS programs across surgical subspecialties have shown decreases in complications and length of stay associated with ERAS, but have also reported pathway adherence rates as low as 65%.[16–22] Given that pathway adherence is associated with improved patient outcomes, it is important to understand the factors associated with ERAS pathway adherence. IS approaches could be instrumental in disentangling this evidence-practice gap by studying the reasons that certain institutions have high adherence rates and introducing those methods in poorly adherent centers.

Another perioperative evidence-based practice is the safety checklist. In 2009, the Safe Surgery Saves Lives study group reported decreased complications and mortality after implementation of the SSC in 8 cities in 8 countries.[23] The SSC is modeled after safety checklists used in high-reliability organizations and includes 19 elements checked at 1 of 3 times during surgery: before the induction of anesthesia, before skin incision, and at the end of surgery.[24] Mayer and colleagues[25] evaluated the impact of SSC compliance on risk-adjusted clinical outcomes. In this multicenter cohort of 5 academic and community hospitals, the investigators discovered the following: (1) SSCs were completed in their entirety in 62.1% of cases, (2) checklist completion reduced postoperative complications by 5.7%, and (3) 14% of complications could be prevented if checklists were fully completed.[25] Levy and colleagues[26] prospectively studied the compliance with all preincision components of the surgical checklist in pediatric surgery. The investigators found that although hospitals reported 100% checklist compliance, checklists were completed fully in fewer than 60% of cases. Finally, Bergs and colleagues[27] performed a meta-analysis of the effect of SSC on postsurgical outcomes, finding a strong correlation between checklist adherence and decreases in postoperative complications. These studies demonstrate that, as with ERAS, improved patient outcomes are linked to intervention uptake and use, and that intervention uptake and use is incomplete. IS-informed approaches can be used to identify implementation interventions that can improve SSC uptake and effective use.

In **Table 1**, we identify additional perioperative IS questions, distinguishing implementation outcomes from intervention effectiveness outcomes.

Perioperative Studies in Implementation Science

Given that IS is a relatively new field with roots outside of anesthesia and surgery, there are few published empiric studies that specifically address implementation, either through identifying factors that influence implementation efforts or through testing implementation strategies (an in-depth review of implementation strategies was published in 2012 by Powell and colleagues[28]). The increasing number of perioperative IS study protocols[29] suggests that this area is a growing area of research. Of the handful of published perioperative IS studies, ERAS is a particular interest.[30–34] **Table 2** presents several perioperative studies published in the past 10 years that demonstrate the application of IS to perioperative research questions.

WHAT THEORIES, MODELS, OR FRAMEWORKS ARE PARTICULARLY SUITED TO PERIOPERATIVE IMPLEMENTATION SCIENCE?

The field of IS relies heavily on theories, models, and frameworks that explicitly describe or explain how evidence is disseminated, taken up, and used. (In the IS literature, there is considerable heterogeneity in the use of the terms "theory," "model," and "framework." A detailed treatment of the differences between the terms is outside the scope of this article, but Nilsen offers an explanation of the differences, with theories including causal relationships and with frameworks generally excluding causal relationships. For the purposes of this article, we use the term "framework" to describe theories, models, and frameworks collectively.)

More than 60 IS frameworks have been used in published IS studies.[35] Nilsen[36] developed a useful taxonomy of IS frameworks: process, explanatory, and evaluative. *Process frameworks* aim to describe or guide implementation efforts. *Explanatory frameworks* tend to be lists of factors influencing implementation, without any explicit statements of causality. Finally, *evaluative frameworks* guide the determination of whether implementation efforts have been effective. Evaluation in this context is interested in the outcomes of implementation. Examples of implementation outcomes include acceptability, adoption, feasibility, and fidelity.[10] We explain implementation outcomes in more detail later.

Table 3 shows several frameworks that have been applied in perioperative settings. Explanatory and evaluative frameworks are commonly used in perioperative IS studies, with the Theoretic Domains Framework[37] being particularly well-represented.

WHAT ARE EXAMPLES OF IMPLEMENTATION OUTCOMES?

As mentioned earlier, IS is focused on facilitating the effective use of evidence-based practices. Implementation outcomes, therefore, capture the use of different facets of evidence-based practice. Enola Proctor and colleagues[10] defined 8 implementation outcomes: *acceptability, adoption, appropriateness, costs, feasibility, fidelity, penetration*, and *sustainability*. Although these outcomes are commonly reported in IS studies, there are few validated measures available for use. In their systematic review of implementation outcome measures, Lewis and colleagues[38] found 104 instruments, but *acceptability* and *adoption* were the only outcomes with more than 10 instruments. Psychometric strength was weak for all but one of the instruments, presenting a challenge to the measurement of implementation outcomes that can be compared across settings.

Table 1
Examples of implementation science questions relevant to perioperative care

Setting	Concept	Evidence-Based Intervention	Implementation Science Outcome and Example Question	Effectiveness Outcome(s)[a]
General surgery	Opioid-sparing postoperative pain control	Multimodal analgesia[67,68]	Acceptability: How acceptable is multimodal analgesia to patients and to ordering providers?	Postoperative pain scores; Cumulative opioid consumption; Length of admission; Return of bowel function
General surgery	Optimization of fluid balance in the perioperative period	ERAS[69]	Fidelity: How well do clinicians adhere to ERAS protocols?	Acute kidney injury; Anastomotic breakdown; 30-d mortality; Readmission rates
ICU	OR to ICU handoffs	Standardization of OR to ICU handoffs[70,71]	Appropriateness: How appropriate is a detailed checklist for use in mixed surgical ICUs?	Information omissions; Handoff duration; ICU readmissions; ICU mortality
Obstetrics	Oral intake for laboring parturients	Permissive oral intake during labor[72,73]	Penetration: How many obstetrics nurses in a given unit integrate oral intake into labor?	Cesarean delivery; Operative vaginal delivery; Apgar scores; Maternal satisfaction
Pain clinic	Use of nonpharmacologic forms of pain therapy	Music therapy[74,75]	Feasibility: How can clinicians incorporate music therapy into patient care?	Pain scores; Emotional distress; Anxiety/depression
Preoperative clinic	PAT for ambulatory surgery	Refraining from ordering laboratory studies in low-risk ambulatory patients[76–78]	Adoption: How many outpatient surgery centers follow PAT guidelines for ambulatory surgery?	30-d adverse event rate; Wound complications
Transplant surgery	Perioperative coagulation assessment for liver transplantation	TEG-guided blood product transfusion[79]	Feasibility: What service will take responsibility for maintaining point-of-care TEG machines in an inpatient setting?	Amount of blood product transfused; Estimated blood loss; Coagulopathy on ICU admission

Abbreviations: ERAS, enhanced recovery after surgery; ICU, intensive care unit; OR, operating room; PAT, preadmission testing; TEG, thromboelastography.
[a] Note: Pure implementation studies would include only implementation outcomes, whereas hybrid effectiveness-implementation designs[43] would include both effectiveness and implementation outcomes. Both outcome types are shown here to contrast the 2 types of study outcomes.

Author(s) and Years	Implementation Concept	Findings
Rycroft-Malone et al,[80] 2012	Comparative effectiveness of 3 implementation strategies to improve compliance with perioperative fasting guidelines	Implementation strategies had different types of impacts on practices, policies, and attitudes, but no difference in food or fluid fasting times.
Russ et al,[81] 2015	Barriers and facilitators of adherence to the Surgical Safety Checklist in 10 British hospitals	Implementation strategies varied across hospitals. Barriers to use included resistance from senior clinicians and problematic integration into workflow. Facilitators included local modifications to the checklist, education and training, and feedback provision.
Gramlich et al,[30] 2017	Strategies to improve compliance with enhanced recovery after surgery protocols in 6 sites in Canada	A theory-informed implementation strategy improved protocol compliance from 40% to 65%. Barriers and facilitators of compliance were linked to multiple factors including patients, individual providers, and organizational factors.

Table 2
Selected published research in perioperative implementation science

WHAT ARE THE CHALLENGES TO IMPLEMENTATION SCIENCE IN PERIOPERATIVE CARE?

There are at least 3 major barriers to the use of IS principles in perioperative research. First, the evidence base supporting many perioperative interventions is weak to moderate, whereas IS assumes the availability of interventions known to be efficacious. Second, IS is a young field as compared with other research traditions. Thus, there are few scientists with the skills to leverage implementation science theory to address issues relating to perioperative research.[39] Third, IS requires the use of mixed quantitative and qualitative measures, but qualitative research remains underappreciated in surgical and anesthesia peer-reviewed journals.[40,41] We discuss each of these limitations in detail as follows.

Implementation Science Rests on the Assumption That There Are Evidence-Based Practices to Spread and Scale

As Glasgow and Chambers[42] explain, IS has relied heavily on a linear model of research in which basic science discoveries precede clinical discoveries, leading to efficacy trials, effectiveness trials, and finally, implementation trials. One problem with this linear view is the necessary time lag associated with following the path from discovery to intervention development to implementation. In perioperative care, which arguably suffers from a dearth of clinical interventions with demonstrated efficacy, IS trials could be years away. In recognition of the delay associated with the traditional linear model of research translation, Curran and colleagues[43] developed the idea of hybrid effectiveness-implementation studies. In these studies, both clinical intervention effectiveness and implementation outcomes are measured. Curran and colleagues[43] describe 3 types of hybrid studies: studies focused on intervention effectiveness that also collect some implementation data (Type 1),

Table 3
Selected implementation science frameworks and examples of perioperative research studies using these frameworks

Framework Name	Original Citation	Perioperative Studies Citing This Framework
Process frameworks		
The Iowa Model of Research-Based Practice	Titler et al,[82] 1994	Haxton et al,[83] 2012
Knowledge-to-Action Framework (K2A)	Graham et al,[84] 2006	Stacey et al,[85] 2015
Explanatory frameworks		
Consolidated Framework for Implementation Research (CFIR)	Damschroder et al,[86] 1999	Lane-Fall et al,[29] 2014 Ament,[87] 2017
Promoting Action on Research Implementation in Health Services (PARIHS)	Kitson et al,[88] 1998; Rycroft-Malone et al,[89] 2002[a]	Rycroft-Malone et al,[80] 2012 Botti et al, 2014
Theoretic Domains Framework (TDF)	Michie et al,[37] 1995	Patey et al,[90] 2012 Gramlich et al,[30] 2017
Evaluative frameworks		
Reach, Effectiveness, Adoption, Implementation, Maintenance (RE-AIM)	Glasgow et al,[91] 1999	Marang-van de Mheen et al,[92] 2006
Realistic evaluation	Pawson and Tilley,[93] 1997	Randell et al,[94] 2014

[a] The conceptual framework was developed by Kitson et al, but the term "PARIHS" was coined by Rycroft-Malone et al.

studies with equal focus on effectiveness and implementation outcomes (Type 2), and studies focused on implementation that also collect data about effectiveness (Type 3). Hybrid designs are still new to perioperative IS, but they have been advocated as promising next steps[44] and have been cited by study protocols.[29]

Implementation Science Is a Young Field

Early IS researchers hailed from fields such as psychology, nursing, and public health, using their skills to develop a new discipline. As we discuss later, there are an increasing number of training opportunities in IS, but there is a necessary lag between these opportunities, the maturation of a research workforce, and substantial contributions to the field. Indeed, as recently as 2001, Goldman and colleagues[45] stated, "There is virtually no definitive evidence to guide implementation of specific evidence-based practices." Although IS is developing rapidly, a 2005 comprehensive synthesis of the published implementation science literature reviewed 2000 articles and found none relating to anesthesia, surgery, or perioperative care.[13] A more recent search of bibliographic databases reveals an increasing number of perioperative IS-relevant articles, but many of these are commentaries,[46] reviews,[47] and study protocols.[29,48] The novelty of perioperative IS represents a challenge to research mentors, potential collaborators, nongovernmental funders, journal readers, reviewers, and editors, who may have limited familiarity with the field.

Implementation Outcomes Include Qualitative and Quantitative Measures

Qualitative research has historically been undervalued in anesthesia[40] and surgery,[41] 2 of the major disciplines concerned with perioperative care research. Why is this important? Many implementation constructs are difficult or impossible to quantify.

Examples include implementation context, implementation climate, feasibility (the extent to which implementation is possible in a given environment given structural, financial, and personnel constraints) and penetration (the extent to which a given intervention has been accepted and used within an organization). Qualitative approaches give rich insight into the settings in which implementation must occur. Without an appreciation of qualitative research methods, then, IS research efforts will not reflect the complexity of implementation in real-world settings.

Qualitative research accomplishes a second important function in implementation research: the characterization of outcomes without validated measures. Ideally, each selected implementation outcomes would have a validated measure, much in the way that the outcome "quality of life" may be measured with the Short Form (SF)-36, SF-12, or other related measures.[49] In IS, however, validated measures are lacking,[38,50] with resultant heterogeneity in the reporting of outcomes. In the absence of validated measures, qualitative characterizations of implementation outcomes serve an important role in characterizing implementation context and the effectiveness of implementation interventions.

WHAT TRAINING OPPORTUNITIES EXIST IN IMPLEMENTATION SCIENCE?

Given that IS is a relatively new discipline, traditional formal training opportunities have been limited.[51] However, in the past decade, multiple formal training programs have emerged. Opportunities for training include training institutes, conferences, internships, fellowships, graduate training, certificate programs, and doctoral study programs with exposure to IS. The Society for Implementation Research Collaboration maintains an extensive listing of IS training opportunities,[52] as does the National Institutes of Health (NIH) Office of Behavioral and Social Sciences Research.[53] Here, we focus on 2 types of training opportunities compatible with part-time study: training institutes and online courses.

Implementation Science Training Institutes

IS training institutes generally consist of intensive in-person experiences meant to immerse the participant in the history, vocabulary, and utility of IS. One of the more well-established IS training institutes is the NIH Training Institute in Dissemination and Implementation Research in Health (TIDIRH, pronounced "TY-derr").[51] The Institute's curriculum includes introductions to dissemination and implementation research principles, theories, and frameworks, as well as sessions dedicated to obtaining IS grant funding. The first TIDIRH cohort trained in 2011, and hailed from psychology, medicine, epidemiology, and related fields. In follow-up surveys, these participants rated the institute highly, and more than 70% had initiated a new grant proposal in dissemination and implementation research within 6 months of the program.[51] As of 2017, TIDIRH continues to be offered at no cost on an annual basis.[39] NIH sponsors additional IS training institutes for specific populations, including researchers focused on cancer studies,[54] mental health, and researchers from groups underrepresented in the biomedical workforce.[55]

Implementation Science Certificates

On a spectrum of training opportunities, certificate courses fall between institutes and degree-granting programs. Certificate programs typically follow a curriculum and offer multiple courses over time, which may be useful to investigators planning to build an IS research portfolio. Some certificate programs are offered online, which may be appealing to clinician-investigators. Certificate programs are generally less costly than degree-granting programs, but offer the advantage of signaling to the outside world that the trainee has met some minimal level of knowledge in IS.

WHAT STRATEGIES MAY BE USED TO FUND IMPLEMENTATION SCIENCE RESEARCH?

IS is commonly conceptualized as part of the continuum linking scientific discoveries to improved health. It is likely this idea that has sparked the interest of various funding agencies interested in maximizing the health impact of their portfolios. In the United States, NIH, the Agency for Healthcare Research and Quality, and the Patient-Centered Outcomes Research Institute are among the funders that have issued multiple calls for funding for IS proposals.

NIH in particular has been an ardent supporter of IS.[56] Since 2000, individual institutes at the NIH have issued grant proposals for dissemination and IS studies.[57] Additionally, NIH sponsors multiple IS training programs, holds webinars about IS, cosponsors an annual conference on IS, created an IS study section (Dissemination and Implementation Research in Health),[58] and continues to issue regular calls for funding IS proposals. The NIH National Library of Medicine hosts the National Information Center on Health Services Research and Health Care Technology, which maintains a listing of NIH funding opportunities related to IS.[59]

Successful grant proposals in IS acknowledge the tenets discussed earlier in this article. Specifically, they accomplish at least 3 tasks:

1. acknowledge the conceptual differences among efficacy, effectiveness, and implementation
2. select clinical interventions with efficacy and, ideally, stakeholder acceptance
3. include an explicit theory or framework that informs study design, execution or analysis

Two recent articles assist investigators in developing compelling and fundable IS proposals.[60,61]

Researchers also may consider using the effectiveness-implementation hybrid designs discussed earlier.[43] Investigators should recognize that the hybrid designs are relatively new and may be unfamiliar to non-IS grant reviewers. Generous citations and explicit outlining of effectiveness and implementation outcome measures may be useful in justifying the use of hybrid designs.

WHAT ARE OPTIONS FOR DISSEMINATING AND PUBLISHING IMPLEMENTATION RESEARCH?

IS studies may be disseminated to 2 types of audiences: specialty-specific and implementation-specific audiences. Given the dearth of published perioperative IS studies, it is likely that specialty-specific audiences may lack knowledge of IS concepts and strategies, whereas IS audiences may lack a deep understanding of perioperative care. There are advantages and drawbacks to targeting each of these audiences.

Specialty-Specific Audiences

There are numerous conferences and scientific journals dedicated to perioperative care, including anesthesia, surgery, and perioperative nursing. Although the barriers to abstract acceptance at specialty conferences may be modest,[62] lack of familiarity with IS may increase the difficulty in getting IS studies published in specialty journals. A Scopus database search in 2017 revealed 46 IS-relevant articles in perioperative care. Only 1 of the top 5 journals in anesthesia or surgery, the *Annals of Surgery*, published more than 1 such article (it published $2^{47,63}$). One strategy to overcome the problem of publishing in specialty journals is to recommend IS reviewers at the time of manuscript submission, which may assist journal editors in finding qualified peer reviewers. Citing and adhering to IS publication standards[64] also may foster the acceptance of IS papers in specialty journals.

Implementation Science–Specific Audiences

IS dissemination opportunities include a dedicated conference, the AcademyHealth-NIH Conference on the Science of Dissemination and Implementation in Health,[65] and a dedicated journal, *Implementation Science*.[6] Although we have stressed that IS is new as compared with other fields, IS has nevertheless matured to include a common taxonomy of terms and theories.[66] IS researchers expect that studies in this field demonstrate an understanding of the difference between intervention and implementation outcomes, and it is conventional to explicitly mention which theories or frameworks have guided the work being presented.

A second consideration is that the field of IS includes researchers from vastly different educational backgrounds, and includes clinicians and nonclinicians. For this reason, special attention should be paid to rich explanations of context that will deepen understanding for readers, reviewers, and editors unfamiliar with the nuances and peculiarities of perioperative care.

SUMMARY

IS is a rapidly maturing field that aims to bridge "the state of the science" with care delivered in the clinics and at the bedside. IS holds particular promise in perioperative care, in which heterogeneity of settings, providers, and patients presents challenges to the application of evidence-based care. As the pressure to demonstrate health care effectiveness and value intensifies, application of evidence-based implementation strategies will become increasingly important in the design and execution of clinical interventions to improve perioperative patient outcomes.

REFERENCES

1. Morris ZS, Wooding S, Grant J. The answer is 17 years, what is the question: understanding time lags in translational research. J Royal Society Medicine 2011; 104(12):510–20.
2. Dearing JW, Kee KF. Historical roots of dissemination and implementation science. In: Brownson RC, Colditz GA, Proctor EK, editors. Dissemination and implementation research in health: translating science to practice. Oxford University Press; 2012.
3. Mitchell SA, Chambers DA. Leveraging implementation science to improve cancer care delivery and patient outcomes. J Oncol Pract 2017;13(8):523–9.
4. Weiss CH, Krishnan JA, Au DH, et al. An official American Thoracic Society research statement: Implementation science in pulmonary, critical care, and sleep medicine. Am J Respir Crit Care Med 2016;194(8):1015–25.
5. Bauer MS, Damschroder L, Hagedorn H, et al. An introduction to implementation science for the non-specialist. BMC Psychol 2015;3(1).
6. Eccles MP, Mittman BS. Welcome to implementation science. Implementation Science 2006;1:1.
7. van Bodegom-Vos L, Davidoff F, Marang-van de Mheen PJ. Implementation and de-implementation: two sides of the same coin? BMJ Quality & Safety 2017;26(6): 495–501.

8. Rogers EM. Diffusion of innovations. 5th edition. New York: Free Press; 2003.
9. Davis D, Davis ME, Jadad A, et al. The case for knowledge translation: shortening the journey from evidence to effect. BMJ 2003;327(7405):33–5.
10. Proctor E, Silmere H, Raghavan R, et al. Outcomes for implementation research: conceptual distinctions, measurement challenges, and research agenda. Adm Policy Ment Health Ment Health Serv Res 2011;38(2):65–76.
11. Institute of Medicine. Best care at lower cost: the path to continuously learning health care in America. Washington, DC: The National Academies Press; 2012.
12. Institute of Medicine. Crossing the quality chasm: a new health system for the 21st century. Washington, DC: The National Academies Press; 2001.
13. Fixsen DL, Naoom SF, Blase KA, et al. Implementation research: a synthesis of the literature. University of South Florida, Louis de la Parte Florida Mental Health Institute, The National Implementation Research Network; 2005.
14. Engelman RM, Rousou JA, Flack Iii JE, et al. Fast-track recovery of the coronary bypass patient. Annals Thoracic Surgery 1994;58(6):1742–6.
15. Kehlet H, Mogensen T. Hospital stay of 2 days after open sigmoidectomy with a multimodal rehabilitation programme. Br J Surg 1999;86(2):227–30.
16. Nicholson A, Lowe MC, Parker J, et al. Systematic review and meta-analysis of enhanced recovery programmes in surgical patients. Br J Surg 2014;101(3): 172–88.
17. Greco M, Capretti G, Beretta L, et al. Enhanced recovery program in colorectal surgery: a meta-analysis of randomized controlled trials. World J Surg 2014; 38(6):1531–41.
18. Hughes MJ, McNally S, Wigmore SJ. Enhanced recovery following liver surgery: a systematic review and meta-analysis. HPB (Oxford) 2014;16(8):699–706.
19. Visioni A, Shah R, Gabriel E, et al. Enhanced recovery after surgery for noncolorectal surgery?: A systematic review and meta-analysis of major abdominal surgery. Ann Surg 2017.
20. Fearon KC, Ljungqvist O, Von Meyenfeldt M, et al. Enhanced recovery after surgery: a consensus review of clinical care for patients undergoing colonic resection. Clinical Nutrition 2005;24(3):466–77.
21. Basse L, Hjort Jakobsen D, Billesbolle P, et al. A clinical pathway to accelerate recovery after colonic resection. Ann Surg 2000;232(1):51–7.
22. Ljungqvist O. ERAS–enhanced recovery after surgery: moving evidence-based perioperative care to practice. JPEN J Parenter Enteral Nutr 2014;38(5):559–66.
23. Haynes AB, Weiser TG, Berry WR, et al. A surgical safety checklist to reduce morbidity and mortality in a global population. New England Journal of Medicine 2009;360(5):491–9.
24. Nishiwaki K, Ichikawa T. WHO surgical safety checklist and guideline for safe surgery 2009. Masui 2014;63(3):246–54 [in Japanese].
25. Mayer EK, Sevdalis N, Rout S, et al. Surgical checklist implementation project: the impact of variable WHO checklist compliance on risk-adjusted clinical outcomes after national implementation. Annals Surgery 2016;263(1):58–63.
26. Levy SM, Senter CE, Hawkins RB, et al. Implementing a surgical checklist: more than checking a box. Surgery 2012;152(3):331–6.
27. Bergs J, Hellings J, Cleemput I, et al. Systematic review and meta-analysis of the effect of the World Health Organization surgical safety checklist on postoperative complications. Br J Surg 2014;101(3):150–8.
28. Powell BJ, McMillen JC, Proctor EK, et al. A compilation of strategies for implementing clinical innovations in health and mental health. Medical Care Research Review 2012;69(2):123–57.

29. Lane-Fall MB, Beidas RS, Pascual JL, et al. Handoffs and transitions in critical care (HATRICC): protocol for a mixed methods study of operating room to intensive care unit handoffs. BMC Surgery 2014;14:96.

30. Gramlich LM, Sheppard CE, Wasylak T, et al. Implementation of enhanced recovery after surgery: a strategy to transform surgical care across a health system. Implementation Science 2017;12(1):67.

31. Nelson G, Kiyang LN, Crumley ET, et al. Implementation of enhanced recovery after surgery (ERAS) across a provincial healthcare system: the ERAS Alberta colorectal surgery experience. World J Surg 2016;40:1092–103.

32. Alawadi ZM, Leal I, Phatak UR, et al. Facilitators and barriers of implementing enhanced recovery in colorectal surgery at a safety net hospital: a provider and patient perspective. Surgery 2016;159:700–12.

33. McLeod RS, Aarts MA, Chung F, et al. Development of an Enhanced Recovery After Surgery guideline and implementation strategy based on the knowledge-to-action cycle. Ann Surg 2015;262:1016–25.

34. Conn LG, McKenzie M, Pearsall EA, et al. Successful implementation of an enhanced recovery after surgery programme for elective colorectal surgery: a process evaluation of champions' experiences. Implement Sci 2015;10:99.

35. Tabak RG, Khoong EC, Chambers D, et al. Bridging research and practice: the use of models in dissemination and implementation research. Am J Prev Med 2012;43.

36. Nilsen P. Making sense of implementation theories, models and frameworks. Implementation Science 2015;10(1):53.

37. Michie S, Johnston M, Abraham C, et al. Making psychological theory useful for implementing evidence based practice: a consensus approach. Qual Saf Health Care 2005;14:26–33.

38. Lewis CC, Fischer S, Weiner BJ, et al. Outcomes for implementation science: an enhanced systematic review of instruments using evidence-based rating criteria. Implementation Science 2015;10(1):155.

39. National Institutes of Health OoBaSSR. Training Institute on Dissemination and Implementation Research in Health. 2017. Availble at: https://obssr.od.nih.gov/training/training-institutes/training-institute-on-dissemination-and-implementation-research-tidirh/. Accessed August 27, 2017.

40. Wijeysundera DN, Feldman BM. Quality, not just quantity: the role of qualitative methods in anesthesia research. Canadian Journal of Anaesthesia 2008;55(10):670–3.

41. Maragh-Bass AC, Appelson JR, Changoor NR, et al. Prioritizing qualitative research in surgery: a synthesis and analysis of publication trends. Surgery 2016;160(6):1447–55.

42. Glasgow RE, Chambers D. Developing robust, sustainable, implementation systems using rigorous, rapid and relevant science. Clin Transl Sci 2012;5:48–55.

43. Curran GM, Bauer M, Mittman B, et al. Effectiveness-implementation hybrid designs: combining elements of clinical effectiveness and implementation research to enhance public health impact. Medical Care 2012;50(3):217–26.

44. Reames BN, Krell RW, Campbell DA Jr, et al. A checklist-based intervention to improve surgical outcomes in michigan: evaluation of the keystone surgery program. JAMA Surgery 2015;150(3):208–15.

45. Goldman HH, Ganju V, Drake RE, et al. Policy implications for implementing evidence-based practices. Psychiatric Services 2001;52(12):1591–7.

46. Brooke BS, Finlayson SG. What surgeons can learn from the emerging science of implementation. JAMA Surgery 2015;150(10):1006–7.

47. Hull L, Athanasiou T, Russ S. Implementation science: a neglected opportunity to accelerate improvements in the safety and quality of surgical care. Annals Surgery 2017;265(6):1104–12.
48. McIlvennan CK, Thompson JS, Matlock DD, et al. A multicenter trial of a shared decision support intervention for patients and their caregivers offered destination therapy for advanced heart failure: DECIDE-LVAD: rationale, design, and pilot data. J Cardiovascular Nursing 2016;31(6):E8–20.
49. Garratt A, Schmidt L, Mackintosh A, et al. Quality of life measurement: bibliographic study of patient assessed health outcome measures. BMJ 2002;324(7351):1417.
50. Rabin BA, Lewis CC, Norton WE, et al. Measurement resources for dissemination and implementation research in health. Implementation Science 2016;11(1):42.
51. Meissner HI, Glasgow RE, Vinson CA, et al. The U.S. training institute for dissemination and implementation research in health. Implementation Science 2013; 8(1):12.
52. Society for Implementation Research Collaboration. Dissemination and Implementation Training Opportunities. 2017. Available at: https://societyforimplementation researchcollaboration.org/dissemination-and-implementation-training-opportunities/. Accessed August 27, 2017.
53. National Institutes of Health OoBaSSR. Dissemination and Implementation. 2017. Available at: https://obssr.od.nih.gov/scientific-initiatives/dissemination-and-implementation/. Accessed August 27, 2017.
54. Washington University in St. Louis. Mentored training for dissemination & implementation research in cancer. 2017. Available at: http://mtdirc.org/. Accessed November 11, 2017.
55. University of California San Francisco CfVPaZSFG. Research in Implementation Science for Equity (RISE). 2017. Available at: https://cvp.ucsf.edu/programs/capacity/rise.html. Accessed August 27, 2017.
56. Purtle J, Peters R, Brownson RC. A review of policy dissemination and implementation research funded by the National Institutes of Health, 2007–2014. Implementation Science 2016;11(1):1.
57. Glasgow RE, Vinson C, Chambers D, et al. National Institutes of Health approaches to dissemination and implementation science: current and future directions. Am J Public Health 2012;102(7):1274–81.
58. National Institutes of Health. Dissemination and Implementation Research in Health Study Section [DIRH]. 2017. Available at: https://public.csr.nih.gov/studysections/integratedreviewgroups/hdmirg/dirh/Pages/default.aspx. Accessed August 27, 2017.
59. National Library of Medicine NICoHSRaHCT. Dissemination and Implementation Science. 2017. Available at: https://www.nlm.nih.gov/hsrinfo/implementation_science.html. Accessed August 27, 2017.
60. Proctor EK, Powell BJ, Baumann AA, et al. Writing implementation research grant proposals: ten key ingredients. Implement Sci 2012;7(1):96.
61. Brownson RC, Colditz GA, Dobbins M, et al. Concocting that magic elixir: successful grant application writing in dissemination and implementation research. Clinical and Translational Science 2015;8(6):710–6.
62. de Meijer VE, Knops SP, van Dongen JA, et al. The fate of research abstracts submitted to a national surgical conference: a cross-sectional study to assess scientific impact. American Journal of Surgery 2016;211(1):166–71.
63. Englesbe MJ, Lussiez AD, Friedman JF, et al. Starting a surgical home. Annals of Surgery 2015;262(6):901–3.

64. Pinnock H, Barwick M, Carpenter CR, et al. Standards for Reporting Implementation Studies (StaRI): explanation and elaboration document. BMJ Open 2017; 7(4):e013318.
65. Chambers D, Simpson L, Neta G, et al. Proceedings from the 9th annual conference on the science of dissemination and implementation. Implementation Science 2017;12(1):48.
66. Rabin B, Brownson R, Haire-Joshu D, et al. A glossary for dissemination and implementation research in health. Journal of Public Health Management and Practice 2008;14:117–23.
67. Andersen LO, Kehlet H. Analgesic efficacy of local infiltration analgesia in hip and knee arthroplasty: a systematic review. Br J Anaesth 2014;113(3):360–74.
68. McCarthy GC, Megalla SA, Habib AS. Impact of intravenous lidocaine infusion on postoperative analgesia and recovery from surgery: a systematic review of randomized controlled trials. Drugs 2010;70(9):1149–63.
69. Zhuang CL, Ye XZ, Zhang XD, et al. Enhanced recovery after surgery programs versus traditional care for colorectal surgery: a meta-analysis of randomized controlled trials. Diseases of the Colon and Rectum 2013;56(5):667–78.
70. McElroy LM, Collins KM, Koller FL, et al. Operating room to intensive care unit handoffs and the risks of patient harm. Surgery 2015;158(3):588–94.
71. Segall N, Bonifacio AS, Schroeder RA, et al. Can we make postoperative patient handovers safer? A systematic review of the literature. Anesth Analg 2012;115(1):102–15.
72. Singata M, Tranmer J, Gyte GM. Restricting oral fluid and food intake during labour. Cochrane Database Syst Rev 2013;(8):CD003930.
73. Vallejo MC, Cobb BT, Steen TL, et al. Maternal outcomes in women supplemented with a high-protein drink in labour. Aust N Z J Obstet Gynaecol 2013; 53(4):369–74.
74. Zhang JM, Wang P, Yao JX, et al. Music interventions for psychological and physical outcomes in cancer: a systematic review and meta-analysis. Support Care Cancer 2012;20(12):3043–53.
75. Lee JH. The effects of music on pain: a meta-analysis. J Music Ther 2016;53(4):430–77.
76. Onuoha OC, Arkoosh VA, Fleisher LA. Choosing wisely in anesthesiology: the gap between evidence and practice. JAMA Intern Med 2014;174(8):1391–5.
77. Benarroch-Gampel J, Sheffield KM, Duncan CB, et al. Preoperative laboratory testing in patients undergoing elective, low-risk ambulatory surgery. Ann Surg 2012;256(3):518–28.
78. Chung F, Yuan H, Yin L, et al. Elimination of preoperative testing in ambulatory surgery. Anesth Analg 2009;108(2):467–75.
79. Wang SC, Shieh JF, Chang KY, et al. Thromboelastography-guided transfusion decreases intraoperative blood transfusion during orthotopic liver transplantation: randomized clinical trial. Transplant Proc 2010;42(7):2590–3.
80. Rycroft-Malone J, Seers K, Crichton N, et al. A pragmatic cluster randomised trial evaluating three implementation interventions. Implementation Science 2012;7(1):80.
81. Russ SJ, Sevdalis N, Moorthy K, et al. A qualitative evaluation of the barriers and facilitators toward implementation of the WHO surgical safety checklist across hospitals in England: lessons from the "surgical checklist implementation project". Annals Surgery 2015;261(1):81–91.
82. Titler MG, Kleiber C, Steelman V, et al. Infusing research into practice to promote quality care. Nursing Research 1994;43(5):307–13.
83. Haxton D, Doering J, Gingras L, et al. Implementing skin-to-skin contact at birth using the Iowa model: applying evidence to practice. Nursing for Women's Health 2012;16(3):220–9 [quiz: 230].

84. Graham ID, Logan J, Harrison MB, et al. Lost in knowledge translation: time for a map? J Contin Educ Health Prof 2006;26(1):13–24.
85. Stacey D, Vandemheen KL, Hennessey R, et al. Implementation of a cystic fibrosis lung transplant referral patient decision aid in routine clinical practice: an observational study. Implement Sci 2015;10:17.
86. Damschroder LJ, Aron DC, Keith RE, et al. Fostering implementation of health services research findings into practice: a consolidated framework for advancing implementation science. Implement Sci 2009;4:50.
87. Ament SMC, Gillissen F, Moser A, et al. Factors associated with sustainability of 2 quality improvement programs after achieving early implementation success. A qualitative case study. J Eval Clin Pract 2017.
88. Kitson A, Harvey G, McCormack B. Enabling the implementation of evidence based practice: a conceptual framework. Quality in health care: QHC 1998; 7(3):149–58.
89. Rycroft-Malone J, Kitson A, Harvey G, et al. Ingredients for change: revisiting a conceptual framework. Quality Safety in Health Care 2002;11(2):174–80.
90. Patey AM, Islam R, Francis JJ, et al. Anesthesiologists' and surgeons' perceptions about routine pre-operative testing in low-risk patients: application of the Theoretical Domains Framework (TDF) to identify factors that influence physicians' decisions to order pre-operative tests. Implementation Science 2012;7(1):52.
91. Glasgow RE, Vogt TM, Boles SM. Evaluating the public health impact of health promotion interventions: the RE-AIM framework. Am J Public Health 1999;89(9): 1322–7.
92. Marang-van de Mheen PJ, Stadlander MC, Kievit J. Adverse outcomes in surgical patients: implementation of a nationwide reporting system. Quality Safety in Health Care 2006;15(5):320–4.
93. Pawson R, Tilley N. Realistic evaluation. SAGE Publications; 1997.
94. Randell R, Greenhalgh J, Hindmarsh J, et al. Integration of robotic surgery into routine practice and impacts on communication, collaboration, and decision making: a realist process evaluation protocol. Implementation Science 2014;9(1):52.

Human Factors Applied to Perioperative Process Improvement

Joseph R. Keebler, PhD[a],*, Elizabeth H. Lazzara, PhD[a],
Elizabeth Blickensderfer, PhD[a], Thomas D. Looke, PhD, MD[b,c,d,1]

KEYWORDS

- Human factors • Medical errors • Safety • Information processing
- Bias and decision making • Performance assessment • Stress and fatigue

KEY POINTS

- Human factors/ergonomics (HF/E) is its own scientific discipline that can be applied to understanding performance in perioperative medicine.
- Humans are not perfect decision makers and are affected by a variety of factors that can greatly harm their ability to perform, including attention, bias, stress, and fatigue.
- HF/E has a unique perspective on human error, and HF/E can illustrate how moving away from blame can enhance safety.
- HF/E offers strategies for undertaking a systematic approach to assessment of work processes in perioperative medicine that can be used to increase safety and wellbeing of patients and providers.

OVERVIEW OF HUMAN FACTORS AND ERGONOMICS

Human factors and ergonomics (HF/E) is a multidisciplinary scientific field that lies at the cross-section of engineering, psychology, safety, and design.[1] HF/E focuses on the relationship between humans and technology at work and attempts to make these human-machine systems safe, reliable, and enjoyable. To accomplish these goals, HF/E considers the design of tasks, equipment, the operational environment, and the training and selection of personnel. Although there has been HF/E work in medicine for decades, only recently has HF/E begun to be integrated on a wide scale

Disclosure Statement: This team has no relationships to disclose.
[a] Human Factors, Embry-Riddle Aeronautical University, 600 South Clyde Morris Boulevard, Office 401.09, Daytona Beach, FL 32114, USA; [b] Department of Anesthesiology, Florida Hospital, Winter Park, FL, USA; [c] US Anesthesia Partners–Florida, Fort Lauderdale, FL, USA; [d] Florida Hospital, Orlando, FL, USA
[1] Present address. 851 Tralfagar Ct #200e, Maitland, FL 32751.
* Corresponding author.
E-mail address: joekeebler@gmail.com

Anesthesiology Clin 36 (2018) 17–29
https://doi.org/10.1016/j.anclin.2017.10.005
1932-2275/18/© 2017 Elsevier Inc. All rights reserved.

into the medical domain. After reports by the Institute of Medicine[2] and more recently by Makary and Daniel[3] highlighting the danger of medical errors and the numerous patient deaths resulting from them, it is pertinent that medical systems' safety is improved. Therefore, this article focuses on the application of HF/E to the medical domain and, more specifically, the perioperative environment. Some of the major theories of HF/E and how they can be applied to understanding the medical work environment are highlighted. The aim is to provide a grounded discussion of the HF/E science within this context and demonstrate the way it can be leveraged to make the perioperative environment as safe as possible. Within each section is detailed a major component of HF/E, and examples are provided from the perioperative environment where appropriate. Finally, suggested remedial strategies based on the various aspects of HF/E discussed are summarized.

HUMAN COGNITION AND PERFORMANCE

To understand work systems, how human beings think and act must be understood. One of the core theories behind how human cognition functions — in other words, how individuals perceive, attend to, and evaluate information from the world — is called *information processing.*[4] Information processing theory (**Fig. 1**) breaks human cognitive capabilities into its constituent parts. These include understanding attentional capacity, perceptual limitations, working and long-term memory storage and recall, and decision-making mechanisms.

Referring to **Fig. 1**, energy from the world — be it light (vision), sound waves (hearing), or pressure (feeling) — enters the various sensory organs and creates a signal. Next, the energy is processed through attentional mechanisms. *Attention* is the process of controlling — either consciously or unconsciously — the limited sensory mechanisms to focus on important information and ignore irrelevant or unimportant information.[5] This information then enters *perception*, which is the interpretation of energy from the world into a meaningful whole and is limited by the filters of attentional mechanisms. *Memory* refers to 2 systems — *working memory*, which is the active cognitive mechanisms, in which information is temporarily stored for use in the near future, and *long-term memory*, which is a repository for the majority of important memories across the life span. Finally, there is *decision making*, which consists of choosing and executing a plan of action based on the attenuated perceptual process and previous experiences.

Human cognition functions by using 2 parallel yet distinct systems for processing information — a perceptually driven system, usually referred to as *bottom-up processing*, and an expertise-driven and memory-driven system referred to as *top-down processing.*[6] These 2 systems work in tandem to lead to conscious experience of the world, yet both are error prone and problematic in certain circumstances. Bottom-up processing uses direct information from the world and is error prone when that information is incomplete — such as when individuals are experiencing high workload, have difficult decisions with multiple potential outcomes, or lack knowledge about a particular situation. Top-down processing uses memory and sums of knowledge to make educated guesses about the world. It relies on experience to make judgments

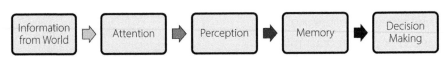

Fig. 1. Basic model of information processing in human cognition.

that can sometimes override direct experiences. As an example, imagine a provider hearing an alarm for the first time that alerts the provider to changes in a patient's health status. This normally would instantly grab attention and is an example of the bottom-up mechanism of cognition. But imagine a situation where the alarm is constant — or is one that beeps regularly on a machine a provider has been using for years. Instead, the provider will likely ignore it, having become accustomed to the noise always present.

The information processing model is important to consider in the perioperative environment because it explains numerous issues arising from the cognitive work of medical professionals. Medical providers are inundated with large amounts of information and must make complex and snap decisions in a work environment full of noise and distractions. Two examples of how information processing can be involved in accidents and the issues that can arise from information processing failures and how they relate to the perioperative environment are highlighted.

Selective Attention

Many failures in human performance are related to attention. Specifically, *selective attention* can undermine the ability to make decisions correctly under moments of high workload or pressure. For instance, a majority of car accidents and incidents involving controlled flight into terrain are arguably caused by selective attention limitations.[1] In health care, providers are inundated with information from electronic medical records (EMRs), colleagues, and monitors as well as alarms, overhead announcements, and a multitude of information from other sources. Therefore, providers are always actively selecting what is important to attend to within their work environment. This has important implications for errors. Can providers be blamed for failures in attention when they are constantly bombarded by various signals from a multitude of sources? Regardless of professional expertise, human beings do not function well in this type of system due to selective attention. It is important for organizations to recognize that all humans have these attentional limitations and to allow for work design that remediates inundating individuals with too much information.

Prospective Memory

Often, providers rely on their memory to keep a to-do list for the work they have to conduct throughout their day. Unfortunately, relying on this type of memory, often termed, *prospective memory* — remembering to remember — can lead to errors in performance. Prospective memory relies heavily on cues — for instance, delivering a drug when a particular alarm sounds — or relies on time — giving a dose of a drug every hour.[7] Both of these processes can suffer heavily from interruptions or off-task activity, leading to major failures in providers keeping to the list in their prospective memory. A common way to counter prospective memory failures is using checklists and other cognitive aids — physical artifacts that act as memory outside of the head. Although little work has directly examined the effects of protocols or checklists on prospective memory performance, much of the work on handovers and transitions of care has found that use of checklists is an effective way to pass large amounts of patient information quickly.[8] Therefore, it makes sense that using these types of tools would remediate the issues that arise from relying too heavily on prospective memory mechanisms.

Decision Making and Bias

Humans can only understand the world through their limited perceptual mechanisms, as described previously. Although it was previously thought that decisions were made by evaluating and weighing each potential option (ie, the normative model of decision making),[9] work by Tversky and Kahneman[10] and decision making scientists over the past 4 decades has instead demonstrated that human decisions are affected by a plethora of biases. Biases are defined as errors in thinking that are based in the limited ability to attend to and process information as well as previous experiences and judgments of the world.

There are numerous biases that can affect work in the perioperative environment (**Table 1**). Many are based in the inability to perceive all information in the world concurrently. Instead, humans make decisions that are based on oversimplified mental simulations of reality,[11] sometimes called heuristics. *Bounded rationality* refers to the state of thinking within the limitations of human perceptual capabilities. In other words, humans attempt to be as rational as possible given limited knowledge, attention, and ability to understand the outcomes of complex decisions. Within the perioperative environment, it is important to consider this bounded rationality when considering blame and the way individuals work. This idea that individuals — acting as bounded rational thinkers — are attempting to do their best in an incomplete and risky world is referred to as the *local rationality principle*. Individuals usually make decisions to the best of their ability yet fail against their best interest.[7] **Table 1** describes some of the most common biases that affect human decision making and offers examples of how these biases may play out in the perioperative setting.

Bias has can be countered in a multitude of ways. Robbins[12] lists some potential remedies. These include staying targeted on goals; seeking information from multiple sources, especially those that might counter values or beliefs; acknowledging and avoiding the formation of causal relationships from random data; and increasing options when making decisions.

STRESS AND WORKLOAD

The health care domain is rife with examples of humans working under high stakes with conditions, such as time pressure, uncertainty, and complex technology; the perioperative environment is no different. Working under stressful conditions can generate negative psychological and physiologic responses, which, in turn, can have both short-term and long-term negative impacts on job performance as well as providers' overall health and well-being.

Stress

The term, *stress*, is used in HF/E to describe the process by which external demands (eg, time pressure, events, and noise) evoke a self-appraisal process in which perceived demands exceed resources, resulting in undesirable physiologic, psychological, behavioral, or social outcomes.[13] **Fig. 2** portrays the relationship between level of arousal induced by stressors and performance.[1] As can be seen, the relationship is an inverted U function. In situations of low arousal (in which the worker is not fully stimulated and bored/not alert), performance tends to be poor. As stimulation increases to a moderate level, performance also improves, until arousal has increased beyond a certain degree, at which point performance begins to drop off.

Over the long term, stress-induced physiologic changes can damage health via effects on the nervous, cardiovascular, endocrine, and immune systems.[14] In addition to long-term decrements in physical health, more immediate impact occurs on job performance,[15] some of these via cognitive effects.[16] Consequently, offering strategies to reduce workplace stressors and/or help anesthesia providers maintain effective performance when under stress is an important area for patient safety.

Table 1
Examples of common forms of bias

Name of Bias	Definition	Example
Overconfidence bias	Individuals are overconfident and optimistic in their abilities.	An experienced anesthesiologist induces general anesthesia without using a checklist and is unable to ventilate the patient because both the CO_2 scrubber and backup airway device are missing. The patient becomes severely hypoxic by the time a replacement backup airway device is found.
Anchoring bias	Individuals attach to initial information and do not update based on more recent information.	An obese patient's oxygen saturation (sat) falls slowly to 90% during robotic prostatectomy in steep Trendelenburg position. The anesthetist, convinced that positioning is responsible, increases positive end-expiratory pressure to 10 cm H_2O and is encouraged that the sat increases to 92%. The anesthetist is then relieved for lunch and the relieving anesthetist replaces the finger pulse oximeter sensor with one on the nose and finds the sat is 100%. At the end of surgery, the finger pulse oximeter is found partially dislodged.
Confirmation bias	Individuals selectively gather information that fits their worldview and ignore or dismiss information contrary to their world view.	An anesthetist requests to have the medication cart restocked between cases and is assured it is done. Toward the end of the next surgery, while the surgeons are finishing a laparoscopic procedure with the main room lights off, the anesthetist draws up the paralytic reversal drugs neostigmine and glycopyrrolate. A couple minutes after giving the reversal, the patient becomes bradycardic and remains completely paralyzed. The anesthetist then discovers that the glycopyrrolate bin was accidentally restocked with similar size and color vials of rocuronium (a paralytic drug).
Availability heuristic	Individuals base their decisions on information that is easily accessible instead of correct information.	An anesthesiologist routinely evaluates cardiac health by asking patients if they can climb a couple flights of stairs without getting short of breath. A healthy-appearing patient answers that he can climb stairs without any problem. After inducing general anesthesia, the patient becomes hypotensive and arrests. After successful resuscitation, a more detailed review of the medical record reveals a recent cardiology clearance note that says the patient is high risk with a severe cardiomyopathy but is in optimal shape for surgery.

(continued on next page)

Table 1
(continued)

Name of Bias	Definition	Example
Escalation of commitment	Tendency to continue with a decision even when it is clearly incorrect	A surgeon persists with robotic assisted laparoscopic surgery, even though there is significant blood loss making it difficult to see what he is doing. He says he is almost done and insists on continuing even after being told that the patient is hypotensive and requiring blood transfusion. He converts to an open approach only after the patient arrests, at which time he discovers a laceration of a major blood vessel requiring vascular surgery intervention.
Hindsight bias	The tendency to believe the outcome of a decision could be predicted after the outcome has already occurred	During an open nephrectomy, a patient starts bleeding profusely and arrests during the 20 min it takes to get blood in the room. The patient is successfully resuscitated but later dies in an ICU. The anesthesiologist blames himself for not insisting that the blood be available in the room before the start of surgery.
Randomness error	Ascribing causal meaning to random events	An anesthesiologist refuses to offer spinal anesthesia to any patient taking herbal supplements after having 1 such patient become paralyzed from a spinal hematoma, even though it is known that herbal supplements do not increase the risk after spinal anesthesia and that this 1 patient probably had spinal arterial-venous malformations responsible for the hematoma.

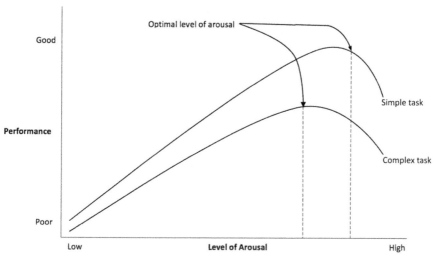

Fig. 2. A graphic representation of the Yerkes-Dodson law demonstrating the relationship between level of arousal and performance during tasks. (*Adapted from* Wickens CD, Gordon-Becker SE, Liu Y, et al. An introduction to human factors engineering, 2nd edition. Upper Saddle River [NJ]: Pearson Prentice Hall; 2004; with permission.)

Workload

Although stressors include environmental as well as psychosocial factors, a prominent stressor is mental workload. The term, *mental workload*, relates the demands of the task to the mental resources of the operator[17] and is an area of HF/E that has a long history of research.[18] The feeling of having "too much to do in too little time" is a simple example of overly high workload and, in turn, may indicate an individual is vulnerable to performance decrements.

Assessing providers' workload level is an important aspect of evaluating the effectiveness of their workplaces, equipment, and procedures.[19] An initial step to identifying high workload situations is to conduct a timeline analysis.[20] A timeline analysis is a task analytical approach to determine overlap in tasks during any point in time.[21] Although task analytical inspections of this nature can indicate high workload exists, examining task time schedules is only 1 aspect of understanding workload. An individual's effectiveness at time-sharing tasks can also be altered by factors, such as extensive experience performing the task and/or automaticity (as described previously) as well as which particular mental resources a task demands (eg, visual vs auditory).[1]

A variety of more in-depth approaches to measuring workload exist and have been well tested in domains, such as aviation and, more recently, anesthesia. Workload measurement approaches include inspection of the speed and accuracy of task performance, adding a secondary task to assess availability of unused mental resources, and physiologic measures (from circulatory, respiratory, central nervous [including visual], and endocrine systems) as well as subjective workload ratings provided by the operators themselves.[22] As an example of the effectiveness of this work, Weinger and colleagues[21,23,24] have had multiple successes using a variety of these techniques in the perioperative setting.

PERFORMANCE ASSESSMENT

Performance assessment, the systematic collection of information to diagnose performance, is arguably the most substantial driver to enhancing the quality of health care and patient safety.[25] It is used to determine the competence of clinical care providers, to provide information to health care consumers, and for quality-improvement efforts.[26] Understanding performance and performance variations, which can only be ascertained through assessment, can serve as the scientific foundation for health policy.[27] Ultimately, performance and the subsequent findings from assessment have an impact on 3 distinct groups: patients, clinicians, and employers.[28] Understanding the impact on these groups becomes complex when considering performance assessment within clinical practice. The complexity inherent within performance assessment is due to the dynamic and interdependent nature of health care[29] and the individual variations within patients.[30]

Although performance assessment is invaluable for advancing quality care, it is not a panacea and must be developed and executed according to the science of learning and psychometrics. According to these sciences, there are several considerations that need to be addressed to maximize performance assessment. The first requirement is to consider multiple levels of measurement.[31] Performance can be measured at the individual, team, department, and even organizational levels. The appropriate level is determined by the knowledge, skills, or attitudes being trained and the type of feedback and remediation necessary to improve performance. The second requirement is that performance assessment should consider processes as well as outcomes.[32] Outcomes represent the end result, and they identify the presence of problems. They alone, however, do not provide any insights into how those outcomes were accomplished, the cause of the result, and what strategies are necessary to achieve a different outcome. Patient outcomes are often cited as the cornerstone of performance measurement[25] but focusing exclusively on such outcomes depicts an incomplete picture. Essentially, it is unknown if the outcome was reached through accurate or erroneous processes. Processes, on the other hand, are more descriptive and diagnostic and offer insights and directions for how to address any behavioral changes. The third requirement is to use multiple sources, techniques, and tools for assessing performance.[33] To elaborate, the source of measurement refers to who is conducting the assessment (eg, supervisor, peer, or learner); the techniques and tools refer to the how and what in regards to devices and procedures used to conduct assessments (eg, surveys, observations, or interviews). Multiple sources, techniques, and tools ensure a more robust and comprehensive understanding of performance. The only way to truly diagnose, deconstruct, and rectify every element of performance is by leveraging an assessment program that heavily considers the science behind psychometrics and learning.

One exemplar study of an operating room performance assessment program heavily scrutinized the aforementioned requirements, conducting a team training intervention and evaluation at a large southeastern community hospital. The assessment program was multilevel and focused on processes and outcomes and included multiple sources, techniques, and tools.[34] Specifically, the research team used a multilevel assessment that focused on trainee reactions, trainee knowledge, trainee on-the-job behaviors, and organizational outcomes (eg, patient safety culture). Within this assessment, the processes included team behaviors (ie, communication, leadership, mutual support, and situation monitoring), and the outcomes were represented as patient safety culture. To ensure that multiple sources and measurement tools were used, the team leveraged surveys that participants completed as well as observations that members of the research team performed.

SAFETY AND ACCIDENTS

Medicine is rapidly evolving, with a current paradigm shift regarding the way it conceives of and reacts to errors. In the field of human factors, errors have been looked at as a systemic issue for decades. In other words, the field of HF/E has treated errors as an inherent aspect of risky systems, instead of as solely the failures of individuals or teams operating within the system. This differs greatly from traditional ideas of error in which individuals are blamed for failures, a way of thinking that is outdated and counterproductive in modern systems and organizations.

There are numerous possible reasons that blame has persisted as an aspect of error management. For instance, blaming individuals means that those blaming are assuming they can understand the cause of an error and prescribe only 1 source of that error — the operator or, in this case, the provider involved in the case. As discussed, ascribing causation to random data is a common bias and is likely behind much of the blame that exists in medicine. But as described previously, understanding causation is skewed by views, experiences, memories, and biases. Blame also moves away from uncovering the operational issues that can propagate and make an organization less safe. Most errors arise from couplings between humans, technology, tasks, and the organizational context.[20] Blaming individuals, then, is not only incorrect but potentially counterproductive: punishing providers for committing errors leads to an organizational culture where there is less of a chance of *error reporting* — an absolutely integral aspect of high reliability organizations.[35] Individuals who fear punitive measures do their best to protect themselves in a system that punishes them.

Root cause analyses (RCAs) have become a common investigative method in hospitals and medical systems. Usually RCAs use interviewing techniques after a medical incident and use these data to discover causal factors leading to the mishap. Unfortunately, even the name itself — *root cause* — is problematic. In almost all accidents there are arguably multiple causes, and assuming there is 1 cause only delays the uncovering of other causal factors. In recent years, RCAs have moved away from their name toward a technique called all-cause analysis. Furthermore, research has called for the integration of HF/E professionals into error investigations to ensure ergonomics and cognitive aspects of work are considered in the management and investigation of errors.[36]

SUMMARY

This article attempts to provide a high-level overview of the field of human factors in relation to perioperative medicine. This is in no way a comprehensive view of the science but it is hoped that enough insight is provided to give clinical teams ideas on where they can start solving issues or changing policies to support safety and better patient outcomes. To tie this information together, some investigators have developed models to represent the multiple moving parts that need to be considered in modern-day health care organizations. One example of this is the Systems Engineering Initiative for Patient Safety (SEIPS) model.[37] The SEIPS model is a representation of the various organizational components — people, patients, tasks, technology, and organizational constraints — that in many ways summarize the entirety of applying HF/E across the health care continuum. **Table 2** presents examples of how these different elements may interact to challenge performance in perioperative settings. Thinking about how HF/E principles apply to safe perioperative care, 3 HF/E-informed guidelines for safety are offered.

Adopt Cognitive Aids and Checklists for Complex Tasks

The use of protocols and checklists has become widespread in medicine. These cognitive aids can be key ingredients to supporting thinking and decision making and should be instituted where a large amount of information is transmitted or

Table 2
Potential issues with human performance in perioperative settings

Issue	Definition	Example
Cognitive fixation	Attachment to previous judgments although new information has arrived that should change that judgment	A provider mis-hears a patient state that she drinks 2 bottles of wine per evening, when the patient actually said 2 glasses. Further diagnoses are based on the assumption the patient is alcoholic.
Plan continuation	Adherence to a plan although cues demonstrate that it is not working	A provider team moves forward with a surgery although the patient was exhibiting some comorbid symptoms that could lead to a poor surgical outcome.
Incomplete or incorrect knowledge, skills, or attitudes	Lack of knowledge, skills, or attitudes pertinent to finding a remedy for a particular situation or escalating error	The certified registered nurse anesthetist had not been part of a code blue in more than 5 y and was unsure of exactly what steps to take next.
Novel technology	Introduction of new tools and technology without appropriate training leads to risks that were not previously in the system and also leads to unexpected information as the system reacts in new and different ways.	The new EMR continually led to delays due to unexpected lockouts, difficulty in finding needed information, and lack of a good user interface.
Dynamic fault management	The need to continue attending to ongoing information and tasks as new tasks stack on top due to system failures	A surgeon accidentally cuts an artery during surgery and needs to manage the subsequent blood loss while also attempting to finish the surgical procedure.

Adapted from Dekker S. Patient safety: a human factors approach. Boca Raton (FL): CRC Press; 2011; with permission.

recorded between providers. The more complex a patient case, the more useful these types of tools can become. Although EMRs have been adopted to fill this role, they come with a set of other problems that have made them difficult to adopt and use, especially in the high-stakes and fast-paced environment of perioperative medicine. Through research and design, cognitive aids can be introduced that work along pinch points that cannot be fulfilled by EMRs alone.

Use Error Reporting Systems

Creation of both anonymous and nonanonymous error reporting systems can greatly enhance organizational mindfulness. The use of both systems is important.

Anonymous systems allow for individuals to report their concerns without having to worry about repercussions or punitive actions. This is especially important for organizations that are going through a cultural change, yet are still relying on the human error model. The nonanonymous system allows for follow-up interviews to garner more information around a specific problem. Allowing individuals to have the option of both creates a culture of understanding and keeps the organization on the path to high reliability.

Enhance the Root Cause Analysis Process

Although RCAs are going through quite a bit of change, they can still fundamentally be useful for understanding errors. Understanding that there are multiple causes is the first step to increasing their effectiveness. Furthermore, integration of HF/E consultants can aid hospitals in understanding potential systemic factors, including equipment and technology failures, issues with team coupling, task complexity, or organizational policy — all potential issues that might be missed by using the standard RCA process.

Summary of Recommendations

Consider the cognitive limitations of health care providers and support staff within the perioperative environment. Although they are experts, they still suffer from the same limitations of any human working in a high-stakes, high-risk system. This needs to be considered in the design of their work environment and procedures and appreciated by organizational leadership. Where applicable, cognitive aids, checklists, and so forth should be used to support the cognitive functioning of medical providers.

Understand that humans work within the confines of bounded rationality and that most decisions are made on incomplete information. Organizations should provide support through decisions aids, safety policies, and cognitive aids to support provider thinking and reduce bias. Antibias training could also facilitate better decision making.

Understand that human error is usually not a satisfactory explanation for why medical errors occur. Instead organizations need to adopt a policy that appreciates the complexity of medicine and values that providers do not want to harm their patients. Human operators (ie, providers) are at the sharp end of the system and usually stumble on errors, not because they are incompetent but because the system is imperfect and risky. Through utilization of error reporting systems and investigations that appreciate systemic factors, medicine can learn about deeper rooted systemic factors and work on fixing them rather than finding a scapegoat and leaving the problem in place.

REFERENCES

1. Wickens CD, Gordon SE, Liu Y, et al. An introduction to human factors engineering. Upper Saddle River (NJ): Pearson Prentice Hall; 2004.
2. Kohn KT, Corrigan JM, Donaldson MS. To err is human: building a safer health system. Washington, DC: National Academy Press; 1999.
3. Makary MA, Daniel M. Medical error-the third leading cause of death in the US. BMJ 2016;353:i2139.
4. Wickens CD, Carswell CM. Information processing. Handbook of human factors and ergonomics. Hoboken (NJ): Wiley; 1997. p. 89–122.
5. Treisman AM, Gelade G. A feature-integration theory of attention. Cogn Psychol 1980;12(1):97–136.
6. Sternberg RJ, Sternberg K. Cognitive psychology. 7th edition. Boston: Cengage Learning; 2017.

7. Dekker S. Patient safety: a human factors approach. Boca Raton (FL): CRC Press; 2011.
8. Keebler JR, Lazzara EH, Patzer BS, et al. Meta-analyses of the effects of standardized handoff protocols on patient, provider, and organizational outcomes. Hum Factors 2016;58(8):1187–205.
9. Edwards W. The theory of decision making. Psychol Bull 1954;51:380–417.
10. Tversky A, Kahneman D. Availability: a heuristic for judging frequency and probability. Cogn Psychol 1973;5(2):207–32.
11. Klein G. Naturalistic decision making. Hum Factors 2008;50(3):456–60.
12. Robbins SP. Decide & conquer: making winning decisions and taking control of your life. Upper Saddle (NJ): Pearson FT Press; 2004.
13. Driskell J, Salas E, editors. Stress and human performance. Hillsdale (NJ): Erlbaum; 1996.
14. Schneiderman N, Ironson G, Siegal SD. Stress and health: psychological, behavioral, and biological determinants. Annu Rev Clin Psychol 2005;1:607–28.
15. Cooper C, Fried Y, Gilboa S, et al. A meta-analysis of work demand stressors and job performance: examining main and moderating effects. Personal Psychol 2008;61:227–71.
16. Rupp MA, Sweetman R, Sosa AE, et al. Searching for affective and cognitive restoration: examining the restorative effects of casual video game play. Hum Factors 2017;59(7):1096–107.
17. Parasuraman R, Sheridan TB, Wickens CD. Situation awareness, mental workload, and trust in automation: viable, empirically supported cognitive engineering constructs. J Cogn Eng Decis Making 2008;2:140–60.
18. Vidulich MA, Tsang PS. Mental workload and situation awareness. In: Salvendy G, editor. Handbook of human factors and ergonomics. 4th edition. Hoboken (NJ): Wiley; 2012.
19. Weinger MB. Human factors in anesthesiology. In: Carayon P, editor. Handbook of human factors and ergonomics in health care and patient safety. 2nd edition. Boca Raton (FL): CRC Press; 2011. p. 803–23.
20. Stanton NA, Salmon PM, Rafferty LA, et al. Human factors methods: a practical guide for engineering and design. 2nd edition. Farnham (United Kingdom): Ashgate Publishing; 2013.
21. Weinger MB, Herndon OW, Zornow MH, et al. An objective methodology for task analysis and workload assessment in anesthesia providers. Anesthesiology 1994;80(1):77–92.
22. Durso FT, Alexander AL. Managing workload, performance, and situation awareness in aviation systems. In: Salas E, Jentsch F, Maurino D, editors. Human factors in aviation. Amsterdam (AN): Elsevier Science; 2010. p. 217–47.
23. Weinger MB, Reddy SB, Slagle JM. Multiple measures of anesthesia workload during teaching and non-teaching cases. Anesth Analg 2004;98(5):1419–25.
24. Weinger MB, Vredenburgh AG, Schumann CM, et al. Quantitative description of the workload associated with airway management procedures. J Clin Anesth 2000;12:273–82.
25. Glance LG, Neuman M, Martinez EA, et al. Performance measurement at a "tipping point". Anesth Analg 2011;112(4):958–66.
26. Landon BE, Normand ST, Blumenthal D, et al. Physician clinical performance assessment: Prospects and barriers. J Am Med Assoc 2003;920:1183–9.
27. Murray CJL, Frenk J. A framework for assessing the performance of health systems. Bull World Health Organ 2000;78(6):717–31.

28. Finucane PM, Barron SR, Davies HA, et al. Towards an acceptance of performance assessment. Med Educ 2002;2002(36):959–64.
29. Norcini JJ. Current perspectives in assessment: the assessment performance at work. Med Educ 2005;39:880–9.
30. Hays RB, Davies HA, Beard JD, et al. Selecting performance assessment methods for experienced physicians. Med Educ 2002;36:910–7.
31. Salas E, Rosen MA, Burke CS, et al. Markers for enhancing team cognition in complex environments: the power of team performance diagnosis. Aviat Space Environ Med 2007;78(5):77–85.
32. Salas E, Rosen MA. Performance assessment. In: Schmorrow D, Cohn J, Nicholson D, editors. The PSI handbook of virtual environments for training and education: developments for the military and beyond. Westport (CT): Praeger Security International; 2009. p. 227–35.
33. Salas E, Benishek L, Coultas C, et al. Team training essentials: a research-based guide. New York: Taylor & Francis; 2015.
34. Weaver SJ, Rosen MA, DiazGranados D, et al. Does teamwork improve performance in the operating room? A multi-level evaluation. Jt Comm J Qual Patient Saf 2010;36:133–42.
35. Wilson KA, Burke CS, Priest HA, et al. Promoting health care safety through training high reliability teams. Qual Saf Health Care 2005;14(4):303–9.
36. Peerally MF, Carr S, Waring J, et al. The problem with root cause analysis. BMJ Qual Saf 2017;26(5):417–22.
37. Carayon P, Hundt AS, Karsh BT, et al. Work system design for patient safety: the SEIPS model. Qual Saf Health Care 2006;15(1):50–8.

Quality Improvement in Anesthesiology — Leveraging Data and Analytics to Optimize Outcomes

Elizabeth A. Valentine, MD*, Scott A. Falk, MD

KEYWORDS

- Quality improvement • Performance improvement • PDSA cycle
- Quality dashboard • Anesthesia quality institute

KEY POINTS

- Quality improvement is at the heart of practice of anesthesiology.
- Objective data are critical for any quality improvement initiative; when possible, a combination of process, outcome, and balancing metrics should be evaluated to gauge the value of an intervention.
- Quality improvement is an ongoing process; iterative reevaluation of data is required to maintain interventions, ensure continued effectiveness, and continually improve.
- Dashboards can facilitate rapid analysis of data and drive decision making.
- Large data sets can be useful to establish benchmarks and compare performance against other providers, practices, or institutions.
- Audit and feedback strategies are effective in facilitating positive change.

The importance of delivering safe, high-quality care has been a core tenet of the practice of medicine since the time of Hippocrates; the dictum *primum non nocere* (first do no harm) is a fundamental bioethical principle familiar to all health care providers. The release of 2 landmark publications from the Institute of Medicine, *To Err Is Human*[1] and *Crossing The Quality Chasm*,[2] brought the issues of safety and quality in health care to the public eye in the early 2000s. Decades before the release of these publications, however, anesthesiologists were already at the forefront of the quality and safety movements. From Dr Ellison (Jeep) Pierce's careful log of "anesthesia accidents"[3] to the early adoption of "critical incident analysis",[4] anesthesiologists have long

No commercial or financial conflicts of interest or any funding sources to disclose.
Department of Anesthesiology and Critical Care, The Perelman School of Medicine, University of Pennsylvania, Hospital of the University of Pennsylvania, 3400 Spruce Street, Philadelphia, PA 19104, USA
* Corresponding author.
E-mail address: Elizabeth.Valentine@uphs.upenn.edu

recognized the importance of evaluating quality in a discerning way. Anesthesiology was, in fact, the first medical specialty to specifically champion quality and safety: first through the creation of the American Society of Anesthesiologists Committee on Patient Safety and Risk Management in 1983, followed by the creation of the Anesthesia Safety Patient Foundation in 1985 and the Anesthesia Quality Institute in 2009.[3,5,6]

The Institute of Medicine defines health care quality as "the degree to which healthcare services for individuals and populations increase the likelihood of desired health outcomes and are consistent with current professional knowledge" and it further refines the definition of quality as having 6 properties or domains (**Box 1**).[7] Measuring quality in health care, however, can be a difficult proposition. The essence of the quality improvement movement is to use objective data to evaluate current performance and use this information to have an impact on positive change.

MEASURING DATA IN QUALITY IMPROVEMENT: DEFINING METRICS

A critical aspect of any quality improvement effort is to determine metrics by which success is measured. It is important to identify appropriate metrics to know if an implemented change represents an improvement over existing processes. Three types of metrics are used in quality improvement.

Outcome Measures

Outcome measures evaluate a desired endpoint of a process. In health care, outcomes measures typically evaluate the clinical impact of a particular service or intervention on the overall health and well-being of a patient or population. Alternatively, outcome measures may assess the impact on other stakeholders, such as payers or the community. Examples of outcome measures include perioperative morbidity and mortality, hospital or postanesthesia care unit (PACU) length of stay, or surgical readmission rates. Anesthesia-specific outcome measures may evaluate incidence of perioperative major adverse cardiac events, postoperative pain scores, or rates of postoperative nausea and vomiting. Outcome measures are commonly reported in large, national databases (discussed later). Although outcome measures may seem to represent a gold standard of quality, it is important to recognize that factors beyond a clinician's control may affect outcomes. For example, Hospital A may have a

---

Box 1
Institute of Medicine quality domains

- Safety — avoiding actual or potential patient harm
- Patient centeredness — meeting patients' needs and preferences and providing education and support
- Effectiveness — providing care processes and achieving outcomes, as supported by best scientific evidence
- Equity — providing health care of equal quality to those who may differ in characteristics
- Efficiency — maximizing the quality of a comparable unit of health care delivered for a unit of resources used
- Timeliness — obtaining needed care while minimizing delays

Data from Institute of Medicine (US) Committee on Quality of Health Care in America. Crossing the quality chasm: a new health system for the 21st century. Washington, DC: National Academies Press (US); 2001.

higher perioperative mortality rate than Hospital B as a result of caring for patients with a higher degree of comorbid conditions, requiring a higher complexity of surgical repair or both. Risk-adjustment methods attempt to correct for varying characteristics between different populations, but optimal risk adjustment is an evolving science.

Process Measures

Process measures reflect on how well a provider adheres to any given step within a defined pathway. In general, process measures reflect adherence to evidence-based, or at least generally accepted, best practices that have been linked to improvements in outcomes. Examples of process measures include adherence to protocols to prevent central venous catheter–associated bloodstream infection, compliance with continuation of β-blockers in patients undergoing coronary artery bypass grafting, or appropriate choice and dosing of antibiotic within 1 hour of surgical incision. Tracking process metrics, not just outcome metrics, helps determine the root cause when outcome metrics are not met as well as cultural acceptance of a given protocol. For example, tracking compliance with a protocol designed to prevent blood stream infections when inserting central venous catheters may identify that the appropriate sterile products are not readily available on the floor. Alternatively, it may reveal that staff object to aspects of the protocol, which may need to be addressed. Having this information is more useful than merely knowing there is an increase in central venous catheter–related blood stream infections. Most of the health care quality measures used for reimbursement and public reporting are process measures.

Balancing Measures

Balancing measures are used to help ensure there are no unintended negative consequences. For example, a balancing metric for an initiative to shorten patient length of stay in the hospital might be evaluating readmission rates after discharge. A balancing metric for an anesthesia initiative to minimize opioid use in the perioperative period might be postoperative pain scores in a PACU. The goal of balancing measures is the ensure that in attempting to affect positive change in one arena, there is no negative impact on other important measures of quality.

APPROACHING QUALITY IMPROVEMENT: DIFFERENT FRAMEWORKS FOR SUCCESS

The basic steps of any quality improvement initiative are to

1. Identify a process with opportunity for improvement
2. Analyze the problem in a systematic way
3. Devise a proposed solution
4. Iteratively reassess performance to determine if the change is successful

That said, there are a variety of methodological approaches to quality improvement initiatives, each of which uses different strategies to achieve the desired result. There is no single correct approach to quality improvement. Three commonly used methodologies in quality or performance improvement are W. Edwards Deming's system of profound knowledge/Model for Improvement, lean, and Six Sigma.

The Model for Improvement

It is impossible to discuss the science of improvement without discussing Deming, one of the fathers of quality improvement. A physicist by training with additional expertise in applied statistics, Deming was sent to Japan in the aftermath of World War II to help correct quality concerns during rebuilding efforts. Deming devoted his life to developing a theory of quality improvement that he called the system of profound knowledge.[8] The core components of his philosophy include an appreciation of the system, knowledge of variation, and an understanding of human psychology. Deming envisioned the Plan-Do-Study-Act (PDSA) cycle, a simple 4-stage approach to quality improvement.[9] This was ultimately incorporated into the Associates in Process Improvement Model for Improvement,[10] which serves as the basic framework for quality improvement endorsed by the Institute for Healthcare Improvement.[11]

The Model for Improvement is a straightforward but powerful tool for approaching quality improvement (**Fig. 1**). The first part of the model raises 3 fundamental questions that are imperative prior to embarking on any quality improvement effort:

1. Setting aims/goals — What is the goal to be accomplished? The aim should be both time-specific and measurable.

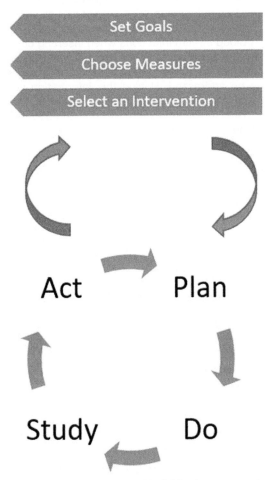

Fig. 1. The Associates in Process Improvement Model for Improvement requires definitions of goals, measures, and interventions before embarking on an iterative quality improvement cycle. (*Adapted from* Langley GL, Moen R, Nolan KM, et al. The Improvement Guide: A Practical Approach to Enhancing Organizational Performance (2nd edition). San Francisco: Jossey-Bass Publishers; 2009.)

2. Establishing measures — How to determine that a change is an improvement? Measures should be quantitative and may be a combination of process, outcome, and balancing metrics to help determine if a specific change leads to the desired outcome, as discussed previously.
3. Selecting changes — What change should be made? Ideas should come from content and process experts who are intimately familiar with the system or process at hand.

Once these questions are answered, the second part of the model is the PDSA cycle. The PDSA is the action component of the model. The goal of this phase is to pilot a proposed change in a real-world setting: first by planning and then by trying the proposed intervention, followed by observing the results and finally acting on the lessons learned, both good and bad, to refine the intervention. A major emphasis of PDSA is the reiterative nature of quality improvement. It is not enough to complete a single PDSA cycle; rather, the intervention must constantly be reevaluated and refine. After piloting a proposed change on a small scale, cycling through several rounds of PDSA cycles for refinement, and verifying the intervention has the intended results, the change may be implemented on an increasingly broader scale (eg, from a small pilot population to the entire operating complex at one hospital to the health system at large).

Six Sigma

The concept of Six Sigma was originally introduced by Bill Smith at Motorola in 1986 and was popularized when Jack Welch incorporated it into his key business strategy at General Electric in 1995.[12] Six Sigma is based in the statistical concept that most results fall into a normal distribution with 2 basic characteristics: an average/mean (denoted by the Greek letter mu) and a standard deviation, or measurement of variation (denoted by the Greek letter sigma). The driving goal of Six Sigma is to achieve perfection or near perfection. Specifically, the philosophy of Six Sigma is to improve quality through the elimination of variation. Driving failure or error to 6 standard deviations (sigma) from the mean equates to approximately 3.4 defects per million opportunities. To frame this concept in a health care context: if the aviation industry accepted the 95 defects per million opportunities (5.25 sigma) level that is the commonly accepted rate of bile duct injury during laparoscopic cholecystectomy, it is the equivalent of accepting 20 commercial aviation crashes each day in the United States alone.[12,13]

Six Sigma methodology uses 1 of 2 conceptual frameworks for quality improvement projects. The first framework is known as DMAIC, which stands for the following key steps: define, measure, analyze, improve, and control (**Table 1**). DMAIC is an improvement strategy for existing processes falling below specification when looking for incremental improvement. The second framework is used to develop new processes where none existed or to incorporate a complete redesign in cases where the existing process is completely inadequate to meet standards or customer needs. The steps in this framework consist of define, measure, analyze, design, and verify. This framework requires the same first 3 steps but focuses on the initial design and validation of a new process. These processes have been validated in complex health care environments to eliminate error and affect change.[12,14,15]

Lean Methodology

Lean methodology was first developed in the production of Toyota automobiles in the 1950s.[16] The lean concept centers on the philosophy of *kaizen*, or continuous quality

Table 1	
Steps in the Six Sigma performance improvement process	
Step	**Description**
Define	Identify the problem to be solved and goals of the improvement project. Obtain necessary support and resources and put together a project team.
Measure	Establish appropriate metrics. Measure baseline performance of the current system.
Analyze	Examine the system for possible areas of improvement.
Improve	Improve the system through implementation of ideas. Statistically validate improvements.
Control	Institutionalize the new system and monitor its stability over time.

Adapted from Martinez EA, Varughese AM, Buck DW, et al. Quality improvement and patient safety. In: Miller RD, editor. Miller's anesthesia. 8th edition. Philadelphia: Saunders; 2015; with permission.

improvement. The lean process evaluates existing processes and adapts them, preserving the steps that add value and eliminating steps that contribute to waste or fail to add value. Lean methodology relies heavily on process mapping, which is a graphic representation of all inputs, throughputs, and outputs of materials or information (**Fig. 2**). Process mapping enables the user to see, at a glance, where waste and non–valued-added steps exist. The 3 enemies of lean design are *muda* (useless work that does not add value), *mura* (unevenness at the operational level, such as fluctuations in quality), and *muri* (burdensome work imposed by poor organization). Any reduction of waste is viewed as beneficial; and, as the goal is continuous improvement, each iterative improvement serves as a new benchmark for further improvement (**Table 2**).

Lean methodology has been successfully adapted to health care to improve quality and efficiency at many institutions. Virginia Mason Medical Center is an example of a health care organization that has fostered an organizational culture focused

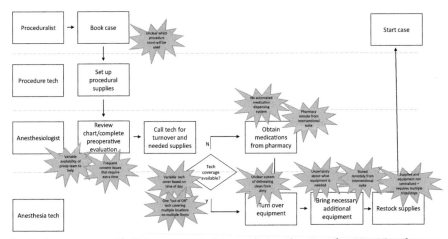

Fig. 2. Process map with Kaizen opportunities outlining the steps for preparing for anesthesia administration in and out of operating room location. (*Courtesy of* Penn Medicine, Philadelphia, PA.)

on innovation and continuous quality improvement using lean methodology.[17,18] Lean methodology has been successfully used in various facets of medical care to maximize efficiency and add value. Examples pertinent to anesthesia care include streamlining computer order entry,[19] minimizing the likelihood of medication errors,[20] and optimizing emergency airway carts.[21] In the last example, lean was used to standardize equipment on a difficult airway cart, scaling down the stocked equipment to only what was needed, which was organized according to frequency and order of use on the difficult airway algorithm. In simulated airway emergencies, this intervention resulted in decreased wasted motion and non–value-added time.

Table 2
Eight types of waste identified in lean methodology

Type of Waste	Description	Examples in Anesthesia
Defect	Products or services that do not meet required specifications and require resources to correct	• Medication administration errors • Readmission for postoperative nausea and vomiting
Overproduction	Making more of something than what is needed or more before it is needed	• Drawing and wasting unnecessary medications just in case they are needed • Ordering blood products without known plan for transfusion
Waiting	Time wasted while waiting for the next step in a process	• Bed delays preventing patient flow into or out of PACU • Waiting for operating room turnover
Nonutilized talent	Underutilizing people's knowledge, talent, or skill set	• Not listening to employees suggestions, leading to burnout • Not using staff at the top of their skill set
Transportation	Unnecessary movement of materials, products, or information	• Central equipment stores rather than storing equipment where needed • Poor layout in patient flow, requiring multiple patient moves
Inventory	Materials, products, or information that is idle or in excess of what is needed	• Excessive stock in storerooms that is not used • Patients waiting to be discharged from PACU
Motion	Unnecessary moment by people due to poor workflow or workspace layout, searching for misplaced items, and so forth	• Poor operating room design layout • Searching for equipment in multiple locations
Extra processing	Any activity that is not necessary to produce a functioning product or service	• Unnecessary laboratory studies or preoperative testing • Duplicative data or entering data into more than 1 place

Adapted from Radnor ZJ, Holweg M, Waring J. Lean in healthcare: the unfilled promise? Soc Sci Med 2012;74(3):365; with permission.

Blended Methodologies

Although the central tenet of all these methodologies is improvement, the PDSA, Six Sigma, and lean methodologies approach improvement with different philosophies and values. Aspects of different performance improvement methodologies can be combined to incorporate different ideals to meet the needs of an individual group or institution. A well-known hybrid of performance improvement methodology is the concept of Lean Six Sigma.[22] Lean Six Sigma combines the 2 methodologies in an attempt to simultaneous improve quality in a data intensive model while eliminating waste.

MONITORING QUALITY: USING DATA FOR ONGOING QUALITY IMPROVEMENT EFFORTS

Data are critical when designing quality improvement initiatives, but the design and implementation of impactful interventions are only the first hurdle. Ongoing monitoring is imperative to ensure continued compliance and continued success. There are a variety of ways to display and utilize data when tracking ongoing quality measures.

Run Charts

A run chart is a simple line graph of a given measure over time, with a horizontal line denoting the median value (**Fig. 3**). Plotting data over time is a simple but effective way to learn about trends, variation, and patterns in data. The main purpose of a run chart is to detect improvement or degradation of a process, and run charts can be used to evaluate the impact of ongoing quality improvement efforts.[23] Run charts have been successfully used for quality improvement efforts in various facets in the perioperative setting, from efforts to improve operating room turnover[24] to detecting opioid abuse among anesthesiologists.[25]

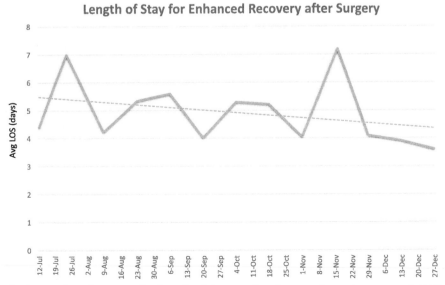

Fig. 3. Run chart demonstrating length of stay over time for an enhanced recovery program with trend line.

Control Charts

Like a run chart, a control chart is a graphic representation of data over time. A control chart always has a center line representing the average value as well as an upper and lower control limit (defined as 1 to 3 standard deviations from the center line depending on process capability), which are determined by historical data (**Fig. 4**). Because control charts define control limits, they can inform on the stability of a process. Within any process, there is inherent common cause variation, or variation caused by unknown factors that results in a steady but random distribution about the average. When the data remain within the upper and lower control limits — that is, when historical experience predicts future performance — the process is deemed to be in control. When 5 or more data points are outside control limits, the process is out of control. This may exist because of a special cause or because of a process breakdown. Either way, it must be investigated to push the process back into control. Special cause variation describes a statistically improbable event and is a signal of a change within the system. An example is special staffing during a holiday or event. Some commonly accepted patterns of special cause variation include any single point outside the upper or lower control limit, 8 consecutive points on the same side of the centerline, or 6 points continually increasing or decreasing as an overall trend. Process breakdowns might occur because a supplier has gone off line or changed their manufacturing standards (**Fig. 5**).

Dashboards

Dashboards are increasingly used in health care as an interactive way to review, analyze, and display performance in key areas (**Fig. 6**). Quality dashboards should help guide decision making in some way: to allocate resources, evaluate quality measures, or steer organizational change.[26] What information is displayed on a dashboard depends on the organizational values and goals. Ideally, dashboards summarize important, actionable, and timely data in an intuitive manner, particularly for users

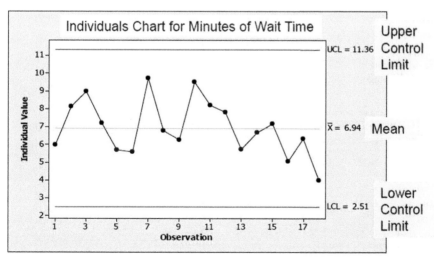

Fig. 4. Control chart evaluating surgical wait time. Mean wait time is identified by the green center line, with upper and lower control limits identified by the red lines. Control charts can help determine whether a process remains in control or if a change has occurred that requires reconsideration. (*Courtesy of* Penn Medicine, Philadelphia, PA.)

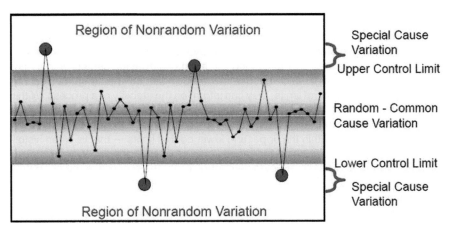

Fig. 5. Control chart demonstrating common cause and special cause variation. Common cause variation is the result of random fluctuations but falls within the upper and lower control limits. Special cause variation can have different patterns but suggests a change in the system. In this example, the red points outside the upper and lower control limits represent special cause variation. (*Courtesy of* Penn Medicine, Philadelphia, PA.)

without analytics experience. In addition to looking at aggregate data, dashboards allow the user to apply filters to drill down on increasingly specific information. Like peeling an onion, peeling back each layer of information may help to understand a process or identify a root cause of a problem.[27]

Big Data in Anesthesia: Registries and Databases for Quality Management

Advances in information and networking technology allow for the rapid collection, storage, and sharing of large amounts of clinical data.[28,29] Although there is no hard definition of big data in health care, the term generally applies to data sets whose

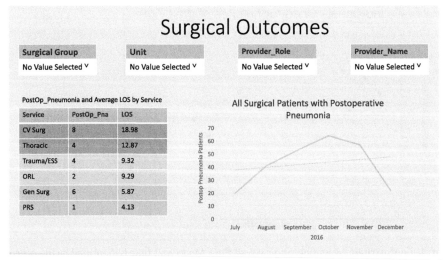

Fig. 6. Example dashboard of surgical outcomes. In this dashboard, it is possible to drill down on surgical outcomes by surgical division, hospital unit, type of anesthesia provider, or individuals. Data are displayed in chart and graphic format.

size, complexity, and dynamic nature require nontraditional statistical tools.[29,30] Big data can be amassed from repeated observations on a local level, such as accruing millions of data points by capturing minute-to-minute physiologic information from an electronic medical record. But although evaluating individual, group, or institutional data alone can help to identify local trends, it does not allow for comparison outside of the group or institution from which the data are obtained.

An increasing appreciation of the potential power of big data has spurred an ongoing interest in the collection of collaborative data in large national data sets. Well-known surgical quality databases include the American College of Surgeons National Surgical Quality Improvement Program (ACS-NSQIP),[31,32] the Society of Thoracic Surgeons Adult Cardiac Surgery Database,[33] and the Society for Vascular Surgery Vascular Quality Initiative.[34] Anesthesia-specific databases include the Anesthesia Quality Institute National Anesthesia Clinical Outcomes Registry,[35] the Society for Ambulatory Anesthesia Clinical Outcomes Registry,[36] and the Multicenter Perioperative Outcomes Group.[37] These large databases have been used to predict operative risk models,[32] set national benchmarks on quality indicators,[33] and evaluate long-term outcomes.[38,39] Participating centers typically receive feedback regarding individual performance against aggregate performance, which can help identify both bright spots in performance as well as opportunities for improvement. Variations in practice, measured adherence to process measures, and outcomes data can be readily identified. A majority of participating centers in the ACS-NSQIP collaborative have demonstrated improved morbidity and mortality outcomes over the course of participation.[40]

AUDIT AND FEEDBACK: USING DATA TO DRIVE POSITIVE CHANGE

Audit and feedback entail providing a summary of clinical performance over a specified period of time.[41] Anesthesiologists, as a group, tend to be both data-driven and competitive. Providing feedback on performance, particularly with objective data, can be highly motivating when used in a thoughtful way. Sharing group performance against national benchmarks, for example, may help engage clinicians as stakeholders in quality improvement efforts. Providing individualized feedback against either national or group performance allows providers to assess their own practice and enact meaningful change. If comparing within groups, it is imperative to blind providers to other individuals' performance data. Feedback may be purely private (data go directly to the provider), or delivered by the quality manager, chairman, or other leadership. The best way to deliver feedback differs between different groups.

Audit and feedback has been associated with improvements in both process and outcome measures of clinical care[41,42] and has been found a more effective tool than both continuing medical education[43,44] and provider incentives.[42] Feedback may be more effective when delivered by a supervisor or colleague, when it is reiterative, when it is delivered in both verbal and written forms, when it includes explicit goals or targets, and when a specific action plan is developed.[41] The importance of continued audit and feedback of performance has been recognized as critically important, because benefits are lost without continued intervention.[45]

SUMMARY

Continuous quality improvement should be the goal for every individual anesthesiologist and group. When undertaking quality improvement initiatives, it is essential to appropriately use data and metrics to understand processes, analyze problems, set goals, and measure change. Data can be used to inform individual providers about performance over time or to compare among providers or groups. Providing clinicians with individualized data can help to drive positive change.

REFERENCES

1. Institute of Medicine Committee on Quality of Health Care in A. In: Kohn LT, Corrigan JM, Donaldson MS, editors. To Err is Human: Building a Safer Health System. Washington, DC: National Academies Press (US). Available at: https://www.ncbi.nlm.nih.gov/books/NBK225182/.
2. Institute of Medicine Committee on Quality of Health Care in A. Crossing the quality chasm: a new health system for the 21st century. Washington, DC: National Academies Press (US). Available at: https://www.ncbi.nlm.nih.gov/books/NBK222274/.
3. Pierce EC Jr. The 34th rovenstine lecture. 40 years behind the mask: safety revisited. Anesthesiology 1996;84:965–75.
4. Cooper JB, Newbower RS, Long CD, et al. Preventable anesthesia mishaps: a study of human factors. Anesthesiology 1978;49:399–406.
5. Stoelting RS. Patient safety: a brief history. In: Ruskin K, Stiegler M, Rosenbaum S, editors. Quality and safety in anesthesia and perioperative care. New York: Oxford University Press; 2016. p. 3–15.
6. Dutton RP, Dukatz A. Quality improvement using automated data sources: the anesthesia quality institute. Anesthesiol Clin 2011;29:439–54.
7. Institute of Medicine Committee to Design a Strategy for Quality R, Assurance in M. In: Lohr KN, editor. Medicare: a strategy for quality assurance, vol. 1. Washington, DC: National Academies Press (US). Available at: https://www.ncbi.nlm.nih.gov/books/NBK235462/.
8. Deming WE. Our of the crisis. Cambridge (United Kingdom): MIT; 1986.
9. Deming WE. The new economics for industry, government, education. 2nd edition. Cambridge (MA): MIT Press; 2000.
10. Langley GJ, Nolan KM, Nolan TW. The foundation of improvement. Silver Spring (MD): API Publishing; 1992.
11. Institute for healthcare improvement: how to improve. Available at: http://www.ihi.org/resources/Pages/HowtoImprove/default.aspx. Accessed July 31, 2017.
12. Mason SE, Nicolay CR, Darzi A. The use of lean and six sigma methodologies in surgery: a systematic review. Surgeon 2015;13:91–100.
13. Sedlack JD. The utilization of six sigma and statistical process control techniques in surgical quality improvement. J Healthc Qual 2010;32:18–26.
14. DelliFraine JL, Langabeer JR 2nd, Nembhard IM. Assessing the evidence of six sigma and lean in the health care industry. Qual Manag Health Care 2010;19:211–25.
15. Deblois S, Lepanto L. Lean and six sigma in acute care: a systematic review of reviews. Int J Health Care Qual Assur 2016;29:192–208.
16. Womack JP, Jones DT, Roos D. The machine that changed the world. New York: Simon and Schuster; 1990.
17. Nelson-Peterson DL, Leppa CJ. Creating an environment for caring using lean principles of the Virginia Mason Production System. J Nurs Adm 2007;37:287–94.
18. Blackmore CC, Kaplan GS. Lean and the perfect patient experience. BMJ Qual Saf 2017;26:85–6.
19. Idemoto L, Williams B, Blackmore C. Using lean methodology to improve efficiency of electronic order set maintenance in the hospital. BMJ Qual Improv Rep 2016;5 [pii:u211725.w4724].

20. Ching JM, Long C, Williams BL, et al. Using lean to improve medication administration safety: in search of the "perfect dose". Jt Comm J Qual Patient Saf 2013;39:195–204.
21. Weigel WA. Redesigning an airway cart using lean methodology. J Clin Anesth 2016;33:273–82.
22. Mills C, Carnell M, Wheat B. Learning into six sigma: the path to integration of lean enterprise and six sigma. Boulder City (CO): McGraw-Hill; 2001.
23. Anhoj J, Olesen AV. Run charts revisited: a simulation study of run chart rules for detection of non-random variation in health care processes. PLoS One 2014;9: e113825.
24. Fletcher D, Edwards D, Tolchard S, et al. Improving theatre turnaround time. BMJ Qual Improv Rep 2017;6 [pii:u219831.w8131].
25. Chisholm AB, Harrison MJ. Opioid abuse amongst anaesthetists: a system to detect personal usage. Anaesth Intensive Care 2009;37:267–71.
26. Buttigieg SC, Pace A, Rathert C. Hospital performance dashboards: a literature review. J Health Organ Manag 2017;31:385–406.
27. Eckerson WW. Performance dashboards. Measuring, monitoring and monitoring your business. Hoboken (NJ): John Wiley & Sons; 2011.
28. Wolfe PJ. Making sense of big data. Proc Natl Acad Sci U S A 2013;110:18031–2.
29. Simpao AF, Ahumada LM, Rehman MA. Big data and visual analytics in anaesthesia and health care. Br J Anaesth 2015;115:350–6.
30. Dutton RP. Large databases in anaesthesiology. Curr Opin Anaesthesiol 2015;28: 697–702.
31. American College of Surgeons National Surgical Quality Improvement Program. Available at: http://www.facs.org/quality-programs/acs-nsqip. Accessed July 31, 2017.
32. Khuri SF, Daley J, Henderson W, et al. The Department of Veterans Affairs' NSQIP: the first national, validated, outcome-based, risk-adjusted, and peer-controlled program for the measurement and enhancement of the quality of surgical care. National VA Surgical Quality Improvement Program. Ann Surg 1998;228:491–507.
33. Society of Thoracic Surgeons. Available at: http://www.sts.org/national-database. Accessed July 31, 2017.
34. Vascular Quality Initiative. Available at: http://www.vascularqualityinitiative.org. Accessed July 31, 2017.
35. Anesthesia Quality Institute. Available at: https://www.aqihq.org/introduction-to-nacor.aspx. Accessed July 31, 2017.
36. The Society for Ambulatory Anesthesia. Available at: http://www.sambahq.org/p/cm/ld/fid=80. Accessed July 31, 2017.
37. The Mulicenter Perioperative Outcomes Groups. Available at: https://www.mpogresearch.org/. Accessed July 31, 2017.
38. Burgess JR, Smith B, Britt R, et al. Predicting postoperative complications for acute care surgery patients using the ACS NSQIP surgical risk calculator. Am Surg 2017;83:733–8.
39. Perri JL, Nolan BW, Goodney PP, et al. Factors affecting operative time and outcome of carotid endarterectomy in the Vascular Quality Initiative. J Vasc Surg 2017;66(4):1100–8.
40. Cohen ME, Liu Y, Ko CY, et al. Improved Surgical Outcomes for ACS NSQIP Hospitals Over Time: Evaluation of Hospital Cohorts With up to 8 Years of Participation. Ann Surg 2016;263:267–73.
41. Ivers N, Jamtvedt G, Flottorp S, et al. Audit and feedback: effects on professional practice and healthcare outcomes. Cochrane Database Syst Rev 2012;(6):CD000259.

42. Chan WV, Pearson TA, Bennett GC, et al. ACC/AHA special report: clinical practice guideline implementation strategies: a summary of systematic reviews by the NHLBI implementation science work group: a report of the American College of Cardiology/American Heart Association Task Force on Clinical Practice Guidelines. J Am Coll Cardiol 2017;69:1076–92.

43. Frenzel JC, Kee SS, Ensor JE, et al. Ongoing provision of individual clinician performance data improves practice behavior. Anesth Analg 2010;111:515–9.

44. Gerber JS, Prasad PA, Fiks AG, et al. Effect of an outpatient antimicrobial stewardship intervention on broad-spectrum antibiotic prescribing by primary care pediatricians: a randomized trial. JAMA 2013;309:2345–52.

45. Gerber JS, Prasad PA, Fiks AG, et al. Durability of benefits of an outpatient antimicrobial stewardship intervention after discontinuation of audit and feedback. JAMA 2014;312:2569–70.

Emergency Manuals

How Quality Improvement and Implementation Science Can Enable Better Perioperative Management During Crises

Sara N. Goldhaber-Fiebert, MD[a],*, Carl Macrae, PhD[b]

KEYWORDS

- Emergency manual • Cognitive aid • Crisis checklist • Patient safety
- Interprofessional team • Implementation science • Quality improvement
- Improvement science

KEY POINTS

- Concepts from quality improvement, implementation science, and improvement research are presented within the context of emergency manual implementation as a nascent area of successful patient safety innovation.
- Stress can cause well-trained professionals, in diverse safety-critical industries, to omit key steps and diverge from optimal management.
- Emergency manuals are tools that can help good teams to perform even better during rare critical events, with widespread dissemination and rising interest in their clinical use.
- The Emergency Manuals Implementation Collaborative (EMIC) provides a central repository for implementation and training resources, links to cost-free downloadable tools from multiple groups, and more at www.emergencymanuals.org.

DEFINING THE PROBLEM

For many rare operating room (OR) crises, such as cardiac arrest, malignant hyperthermia (MH), or local anesthetic systemic toxicity, there are stacks of published literature on optimal management. Yet, even expert clinicians often omit or delay key actions, with detrimental impacts on patient morbidity and mortality.[1] In multiple simulation-based

---

Disclosure Statement: The authors have nothing to disclose.
[a] Department of Anesthesiology, Perioperative and Pain Medicine, Stanford University School of Medicine, 300 Pasteur Drive, Room H3580, Stanford, CA 94305-5640, USA; [b] Department of Experimental Psychology, University of Oxford, Tinbergen Building, 9 South Parks Road, Oxford OX1 3UD, UK
* Corresponding author.
E-mail address: saragf@stanford.edu

Anesthesiology Clin 36 (2018) 45–62
https://doi.org/10.1016/j.anclin.2017.10.003
1932-2275/18/© 2017 The Authors. Published by Elsevier Inc. All rights reserved.

anesthesiology.theclinics.com

studies, correct performance of key actions during crises dramatically increased when emergency manuals (EMs), crisis checklists, or cognitive aids were used.[2–4]

This article examines how the principles of implementation science and quality improvement have been applied in the development, testing, and systematic implementation of EMs in perioperative care. We present evidence from simulation-based OR studies; reflect on related experiences in other safety-critical industries, such as aviation; and describe a conceptual framework for implementation along with data from early clinical uses and implementation efforts. We also explore the practical, organizational, and social processes that influence implementation, and conclude with reflections on the future role of EM implementation as a model for other quality improvement and implementation science efforts.

TERMINOLOGY

EMs are context-relevant sets of cognitive aids, such as crisis checklists, that are intended to provide professionals with key information for managing rare emergency events. Synonyms and related terms include crisis checklists; emergency checklists; and cognitive aids, a much broader term, although often also used to describe tools for use during emergency events specifically.

Throughout this article we use the term "emergency manual," except when referring generically to any of these as tools or when describing a specific study with its own terminology. However, the previously mentioned synonyms could be used interchangeably.

ENABLING TOOLS

EMs are intended as educational and clinical tools. They represent highly condensed repositories of practical knowledge that must be carefully designed and that require training to enable rapid use under conditions of significant pressure. EMs also seek to facilitate effective teamwork and decision making within the collective practice of health care professionals.

EMs are intended to be symbiotic adjuncts with, rather than replacements for, good preparation, teamwork, and judgment, and EM use should never precede necessary immediate actions, such as chest compressions for a pulseless patient. Their intended use begins only once resources allow; either sufficient help is available for synchronous use from the beginning of a crisis, or initial clinical actions are already underway. **Fig. 1** shows EMs being used during simulated critical events.

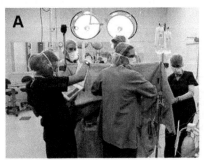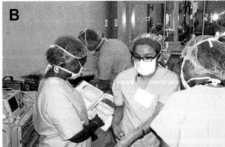

Fig. 1. Emergency manual use by anesthesiologists during simulated critical events. (*A*) In resident course on Anesthesia Crisis Resource Management at Stanford University School of Medicine. (*B*) In simulation instructor course at Stanford University School of Medicine. ([*A*] *Courtesy of* D. Gaba, with permission; [*B*] S. Goldhaber-Fiebert, with permission.)

EMERGENCY MANUALS IMPLEMENTATION COLLABORATIVE: RESOURCES AND REACH

For decades, Advanced Cardiac Life Support cards and MH posters were the only readily available cognitive aids for OR clinical use during critical events. Now, the Emergency Manuals Implementation Collaborative (EMIC) provides a central location for links to multiple cost-free downloadable tools, and implementation and training resources for any such tool, and relevant published literature (www.emergencymanuals.org/).[5]

There has been broad dissemination of multiple tools since EMIC began in 2012: greater than 80,000 combined downloads of various English-language tools; translations of these tools into other languages have also spread rapidly (eg, >200,000 downloads of Chinese versions alone[6]); many downloaders state they shared the tools with colleagues at their local institutions, implying broader dissemination; and these tools seem to be filling a need, with active interest in the concept. **Figs. 2–4.** show examples from multiple available tools (at end of the article, given size). Although dissemination to date has been promising, downloading is only an initial step toward systematic implementation and effective clinical use.

LEARNING FROM OTHER INDUSTRIES

Safety-critical industries, such as aviation and nuclear power, actively use EMs and similar tools in their operational activities. Professionals in these industries undertake regular training in the management of emergency scenarios and the use of EMs, and rely on EMs in actual emergency events. Relying on memory alone is a risky strategy in time-pressured, high-stakes emergency situations.

Even well-trained and highly experienced professionals are often not able to retrieve and deploy detailed knowledge under stress, and this is particularly the case for rarely used information.[7] This is equally the case in health care. Common errors during management of simulated OR critical events include diagnostic and therapeutic cognitive errors,[8] and cognitively recalling but never completing an action. One of the reasons for the latter is a failure of prospective memory, forgetting to do something you intended to do. Prospective memory is particularly vulnerable to interruptions, which are frequent during crises.[9] The use of EMs, combined with good training, teamwork, and judgment, is beginning to address these issues.[10–12] Still, rigorous larger studies using mixed quantitative and qualitative methods are needed to further understand and guide appropriate EM clinical implementation and use.

EMERGENCY MANUALS: A HISTORY AND A FRAMEWORK

The development and use of EMs builds on a century of related efforts to improve patient safety. The first known mention of EMs was almost a century ago. In 1924, Dr Wayne Babcock (the surgeon famous for Babcock forceps) wrote "If a response is not instantly obtained by simple measures [ie, immediate actions], a fixed emergency routine [ie, an EM or similar tool], posted on the walls of every operating room [ie, accessible where needed], and drilled into every member of the staff should be enforced" [ie, prior training along with a culture of expected use].[13] An in-depth history of simulation, teamwork training, cognitive aids, and checklists is beyond the scope of this article, but further background in the literature is provided.[9,14–19]

For many years, Advanced Cardiac Life Support cards and MH posters were the only readily available cognitive aids for OR critical events. Early work by Gaba and coworkers,[9] Howard and coworkers,[14] and Runciman and Merry[20] developed succinct content for cognitive aids spanning a wider range of critical events. In the past few years, development work by multiple groups in parallel has provided cost-free access to several OR EMs, which are designed for use during crises and each linked via the EMIC Web site (see **Figs. 2–4**).[21] At the same time, Gawande's popular book *The Checklist Manifesto*,[17] along with multiple health care implementation efforts and studies of routine checklists,[22,23] spread the concept that human cognition is fallible and increased the receptivity of clinicians to the potential benefits of EMs.

When Babcock made his proposal more than 90 years ago, the health care community was seemingly not yet ready to accept and embrace the utility of EMs. In contrast, the message is now spreading quickly. There is also an increasing recognition that all cognitive aid use exists within the broader context of teamwork and dynamic decision-making skills (**Fig. 5**). Gaba and Pierce[24] have provided a detailed description of how EMs developed within anesthesiology from a rich broader history of cognitive aids and checklists, highlighting contributions of multiple groups globally.

A conceptual framework for clinical implementation of EMs has been developed and can be applied to any field of health care. It defines four key elements that enable effective implementation (**Fig. 6**).[25] In practice, these elements overlap and interact nonlinearly[26]:

1. *Create* (often by locally customizing an existing tool): Refine EM content and design for the specific practical tool to be implemented.
2. *Familiarize*: Train clinicians for EM use, including why, when, and how to apply in practice.
3. *Use* clinically: Put into practice, ensuring accessibility in all needed locations and supporting all appropriate team-based interactions, such as triggering EM use and enabling a "reader" role.

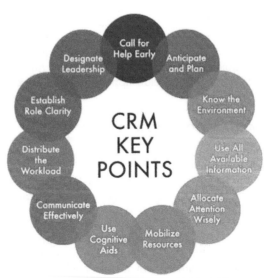

Fig. 5. Crisis resource management teamwork and dynamic decision-making interacting skills, including "use cognitive aids." (*Courtesy of* S. Goldhaber-Fiebert, K. McCowan, K. Harrelson, R. Fanning, S. Howard, D. Gaba; with permission.)

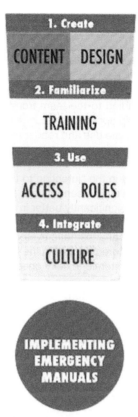

Fig. 6. Four vital elements for implementing emergency manuals. (*Courtesy of* S. Goldhaber-Fiebert, S. Howard; with permission.)

4. *Integrate*: Embed EM use into local culture and professional practice, shaping clinician expectations, attitudes, and behavior as described in the fields of implementation science and improvement research.

As with other improvement efforts in health care, early experiences show that addressing these vital elements is greatly enabled by leadership engagement, local champions, and interprofessional implementation teams.[27,28] Simulation studies and early clinical implementation have made it clear that having a tool available to implement is a necessary start, but is vastly insufficient for enabling effective use.

SIMULATION-BASED STUDIES OF EMERGENCY MANUALS

One of the most important ways of enabling effective clinical use of EMs involves engaging clinicians in an immersive fashion to demonstrate the rationale of why to use EMs and the practical details of how to use them. There is now a decade of studies examining whether the use of EMs helps clinicians, or teams, perform better during simulated OR crises. The preponderance of the data points to "yes," although there are clearly important nuances involved in how to best use these tools. A relevant subset of these simulation studies is described here.

In a 2006 observational study of anesthesia residents managing simulated MH cases, Harrison and colleagues[2] found a positive correlation between the frequency of MH cognitive aid use and appropriate treatment of MH. Burden and colleagues[29] found that most anesthesia and obstetrics residents did not use easily accessible cognitive aids, and proceeded to omit key actions during management of MH and obstetric cardiac arrest simulated scenarios. However, when a medical student "reader" was explicitly charged with reading to the team from the cognitive aid, key actions were then performed and the help appreciated, suggesting the question of how teams can be trained to trigger appropriate use and reader roles themselves. Bould and colleagues[30] found no difference in management of neonatal resuscitation with and without a cognitive aid poster, but importantly subjects were not familiar with the poster before the scenario and most in the "intention to treat" intervention group did not use it frequently, that is, if it is not used it cannot help. Neal and colleagues[3] found that anesthesia residents performed significantly better in managing a surprise scenario of local anesthetic systemic toxicity when randomized to have access to a previously introduced, therefore familiar, local anesthetic systemic toxicity checklist versus not having access to the checklist. Moreover, within the intervention group, the residents who used the local anesthetic systemic toxicity checklist more frequently performed even better.

Arriaga and colleagues[4] studied interprofessional OR teams managing eight different OR crises. Each team was randomly assigned to managing half of the events with, and half without, crisis checklists, serving as their own control subjects. The teams were familiarized with the crisis checklists concept and format, although not the specific events. When crisis checklists were available versus not, 6% versus 23% of key management steps were missed, signifying a large improvement in event management.

Marshall[31] broadly reviewed cognitive aid literature from a variety of settings and also discussed the potential impact of design factors for cognitive aids in health care. Subsequently, Marshall's group conducted multiple simulation studies to understand the impacts of cognitive aid designs and use on team functioning and nontechnical teamwork skills.[32,33] Watkins and colleagues[34,35] studied paper and electronic versions of EMs in simulated settings, where residents were briefly familiarized with both EM formats, but had not typically used EMs previously. They found that about a third of participants did not use the assigned tool when confronted with an applicable critical event, that paper tended to be preferred over electronic, and that both formats had only limited impacts on performance. This suggests that factors beyond the simple use of a cognitive aid are important, such as more extensive training on when and how to use such tools, and tool design. Goldhaber-Fiebert and Howard[25] put the health care simulation literature into context with findings from other safety-critical industries and decades of iterative simulation-based development and testing, proposing the four-element implementation framework described previously.

EARLY CLINICAL IMPLEMENTATIONS AND TRAININGS: DATA AND FURTHER RESOURCES

Neily and colleagues[36] surveyed Veteran Health Administration (VHA) anesthesia professionals 6 months after national VHA implementation of a 14-event clinical cognitive aid for OR critical events, which was initiated at the Palo Alto VHA and drew on prior work from the book *Crisis Management in Anesthesiology*.[9] Of the respondents, 87% knew it existed, half had used it as a reference, and 7% had used it during a crisis. All crisis users believed it was helpful and had used it previously as a reference, which likely improved their familiarity with and awareness of the tool. Training varied across VHA sites, and crisis users were more likely to have received formal training.[36] Although 7% may not sound like much, the relevant denominator of applicable critical events in 6 months since implementation is not known and likely is itself small with only a subset of respondents even encountering an applicable opportunity.

Following recent widespread cost-free dissemination of Ariadne Lab's crisis checklists,[37] Stanford emergency manual for perioperative critical events,[38] and Society for Pediatric Anesthesia's critical events checklists,[39] there have been case reports,[10,11] case series of uses,[12] and many personal accounts of effective clinical uses of EMs during clinical critical events (see **Figs. 2–4** for example pages from these tools). The common emerging themes from clinical uses of EMs to date include:

- Importance of EM accessibility and familiarity
- Value of interprofessional immersive trainings (with high- or low-tech simulations)
- The need for someone on the team to suggest or trigger use
- Helpfulness of a reader role, separate from event leader, when resources allow
- The potential for EMs to improve team communication
- The potential for EMs to improve patient management actions

Clearly, there are challenges to impact and generalizability when single case uses are described individually. However, the multiple early reports do suggest that these tools are being used clinically and that at least some clinicians have found them to be helpful for patient care, underscoring the need for more formal mixed-methods research on clinical implementation and use of EMs.

Clinical implementation research for EMs is nascent. In a Stanford mixed-methods survey study of early clinical uses, 19 (45%) respondent residents had used an EM during a clinical perioperative critical event in the 15 months since implementation.[12] Most users believed the EM helped their teams deliver better care to their patient, and none believed it hurt or distracted from care. There was a wide variety of event types for which EMs were used. Residents also reported that OR safety culture supporting appropriate cognitive aid use improved since implementation and that the most impactful exposures were mannequin-based simulations of critical events coupled with self-review.

A study of OR staff trainings for EMs and teamwork skills showed increased awareness of, familiarity with, and intention to use EMs in the future, using in situ low-tech simulation during brief but widespread division-based trainings.[40] The full training curriculum, instructor guide, and handouts are available for local use or adaptation.[41] Multiple groups have published or shared video-based materials for why, how, and when to effectively use EMs.[42–44]

As more institutions are pursuing EM implementation locally, they are finding important factors to support success include leadership engagement, local champions, interprofessional implementation teams, broader culture of safety and quality improvement efforts, and local customization at least for key phone numbers and conformity with local policies.[28]

MAKING MANUALS WORK: IMPLEMENTATION AND IMPROVEMENT

Implementing EMs is a complex process that encounters difficult practical challenges. Complex, socially adaptive work is required to integrate EMs into frontline practice by changing collective knowledge, attitudes, and behaviors; this work represents a significant challenge and a core component of EM use. Historically, efforts to develop and implement various cognitive aids in health care have followed a common pattern.

They have started with an intense focus on the design and immediate use of the tool itself, and then gradually broadened and deepened to consider the social and cultural challenges that arise when attempting to reshape professional practice and reorganize coordinated action in complex health care institutions.[45]

Because EMs often aim to facilitate effective teamwork, decision making, and management actions, close attention must be paid to the design and customization of the tools; the knowledge and skills of individual clinicians; the collective attitudes, norms, and beliefs; and the organizational processes and systems that all shape professional behavior in real-world settings. A range of research in this area has clear implications for implementing EMs and other safety innovations, spanning four interrelated areas: (1) establishing a problem to motivate changes in professional practice, (2) local ownership, (3) organizational systems, and (4) customization (**Table 1**).

Establishing a Problem

First, changing professional practice depends on professionals accepting that practice should and can be changed. The "work before the work" requires defining and agreeing that there is a problem—and an opportunity to improve.[46] For EMs, this often involves establishing that human fallibility is universal; that fallibility can have particularly detrimental effects in emergencies; and that there are supportive tools, such as EMs, that can address these problems. Demonstrating this through the use of locally relevant data, supplemented by immersive experiences or engaging stories can be a powerful way of preparing professionals for the need to change practice.[47] Establishing that there is a problem that can be addressed, the rationale for why change is needed, coupled with a sense of urgency, is the first step in building the social receptivity to change.

Local Ownership

Second, a sense of ownership of a new intervention is vital to successful uptake.[48,49] This is fostered by local individuals championing a particular intervention, such as a

Table 1
Social and organizational processes underpinning implementation of safety innovations, such as emergency manuals

Social and Organizational Process	Approach to Implementation
Establishing a problem	Building agreement and acceptance that there is a gap between current and desired outcomes, which EMs can help address. This process is often facilitated by presenting a blend of data, immersive experiences, and stories from respected thought leaders.
Local ownership	Fostering a sense of local ownership and buy-in by creating an interprofessional team that leads the implementation effort and by identifying respected champions who model engagement with EMs.
Organizational systems	Reorganizing local systems to ensure resources are provided, equipment is in place, incentives are aligned, and training is routinized to enable EM use.
Customization and improvement	Supporting appropriate customization and adaptation of EM to fit with local requirements, and careful consideration of interactions with existing local processes of care delivery. *Pearl: Preserve the core essence of the innovation, while adapting the periphery of the innovation to better fit the local setting.*

new EM. However, champions need to be well-respected and seen as legitimate within the professional group they are seeking to influence; this may necessitate multiple inter-professional champions. Such champions need to demonstrate the value of the intervention in their own behavior, and that of other respected role models, and challenge inappropriate behavior.[50] Local data and clinical stories of uses, for example, within case conferences or morbidity and mortality presentations, are powerful ways of illustrating local success. It is also important that, in championing an intervention like newly introduced EMs, debate and challenge is encouraged about what works and why, and what does not work and can be improved. This can encourage openness and broad ownership, with engagement of critics rather than alienation. These elements are all essential for the widespread implementation of EMs that need to be owned, understood, and shared by most clinicians in a professional practice. Building this sense of collective ownership, and peer-support and peer-accountability, can provide a strong driver to the social adoption of new practices and tools.[47,51]

Organizational Systems

Third, EMs need to be aligned with and supported by local organizational systems and resources, and embedded in collective practice. Like any tool for supporting and organizing coordinated action, EMs are dependent on the skills and training of those who are responding to an emergency, and the resources and equipment available and broader organizational mechanisms that support frontline professionals. The introduction of EMs can act as a catalyst to improve and restructure broader organizational systems prompting helpful changes to the way other processes are organized.[52] In some cases, implementing an EM may represent a process of standardization, which can reveal gaps in and intersect with other processes, such as the reliable provision of relevant equipment or coordination among multiple professions in preventing or responding to crises. Equally, EMs are most effective when they are part of usual and expected, collective practice for crisis management. This requires effective familiarization and training, which in turn requires organizational resources and systems to support that training.[53] Interprofessional simulations or drills can help increase familiarity with the tool and the tasks required; they can also, critically, increase trust and improve interprofessional communication, common weak points in preventing or managing emergencies, with potentially far reaching benefits.[50]

Customization and Improvement

Fourth, adaptation and the continual improvement of EMs and similar tools is important so that they are customized appropriately to the local setting. This customization process can also broaden engagement and a local sense of ownership of the tool, making it more likely that it will be incorporated into usual practice. Engaging in customization requires developing clarity regarding which elements of a tool and its implementation are core and essential, and which peripheral elements benefit from local customization.[54] For EMs, customization often involves adding or adapting one or more of the following local attributes: emergency telephone numbers, specific response to massive hemorrhage, formulary medication names and dosing, and available equipment or resources.

There are also risks that local customizations might inadvertently reduce the effectiveness of a tool, such as by altering essential elements of its design, introducing typographic errors, or adding so much content that it is less readable. As such, it is important that local customization is properly managed and reviewed. Rigorous processes have been established in other sectors, such as aviation, where master checklists are produced by equipment manufacturers and approved by national regulators; then, each operator has dedicated employees with expertise in checklist development for locally adding or tailoring certain elements according to their own systems and processes.[55] High-reliability organizations, such as nuclear power stations and airlines, regularly review their emergency checklists, updating or improving them when necessary through processes of ongoing testing, advancements in the field, incident reporting, and input from front-line professionals.[56,57] This ensures that frontline staff retain a sense of ownership, and harnessing real-world uses and simulation trainings as opportunities to also test the tool against the demands of reality.[51,58]

EMERGENCY MANUAL FUTURES: DISCUSSION AND IMPLICATIONS

Perioperative medicine has reached a tipping point in enabling effective use of EMs to help teams deliver better patient care during critical events. The evidence base from simulation-based health care studies and from other safety-critical, high-reliability industries has shown a need to more reliably manage crises. EMs can fill this need when used effectively. Several cost-free tools are now widely available for OR clinical settings, along with detailed implementation and training resources.

The findings described here combine to suggest a useful role for EMs in helping clinical health care teams deliver optimal care to patients during critical events. Many important implementation challenges and research questions are worthy of further exploration. Among the next priorities regarding OR EMs are to describe dissemination, adoption, implementation, and clinical uses; assess barriers and facilitators for EM implementation and use; further share effective implementation, training, and use strategies; and actively seek out and mitigate any potential harms.

The implementation of perioperative EMs also provides a potentially powerful broader model of how quality improvement efforts can interact synergistically with implementation science. Many of the transferrable lessons involve the important roles of the following factors: leadership support, local champions, training and simulation, interprofessional involvement, and combining scientific data and immersive experiences to influence practice. Almost all safety interventions in health care represent complex practical, social, and adaptive problems, involving the intersections of individual clinicians' knowledge, skills, and attitudes, broader teamwork and communication, systems processes, and local cultures. It is therefore unsurprising that improvement efforts also require complex and adaptive approaches to be successful. The lessons from the implementation of EMs described here, integrating contextually sensitive and socially adaptive approaches early in the process, are likely applicable to effectively implementing many other safety interventions in anesthesiology and perioperative care.

ACKNOWLEDGMENTS

Many individuals, teams, and institutions have contributed to the development, testing, clinical implementation, use, and study of EMs. In particular, the authors thank the Stanford Emergency Manual team (Stanford Anesthesia Cognitive Aid Group), Ariadne Lab's Project Check, and The Society for Pediatric Anesthesia's Quality and Safety Committee for sharing the cost-free tools they each developed along with resources for using them well; EMIC steering committee for gathering EM tools, implementation, and training resources in one location (www.emergencymanuals. org); and the many clinicians who have shared their experiences and given feedback to improve design, training, implementation, and use of EMs. S.N. Goldhaber-Fiebert is grateful to Foundation for Anesthesia Education and Research (FAER) for a Research in Education Grant that is enabling further research in this area.

A

Society for Pediatric Anesthesia
education • research • patient safety

PediCrisis

CRITICAL EVENTS CARDS

Call for help!	
Code Team	_____
PICU	_____
Fire	_____
Overhead STAT	_____
ECMO	_____

Notify surgeon.

Revision February 8, 2017

Air Embolism	2
Anaphylaxis	3
Anterior Mediastinal Mass	4
Bradycardia	5
Cardiac Arrest	6–8
Difficult Airway	9
Fire: Airway / OR	10–11
Hyperkalemia	12
Hypertension	13
Hypotension	14
Hypoxia	15
Intracranial Pressure	16
Local Anesthetic Toxicity	17
Loss of Evoked Potentials	18
Malignant Hyperthermia	19
Myocardial Ischemia	20
Pulmonary Hypertension	21
Tachycardia	22
Tension pneumothorax	23
Transfusion & Reactions	24–25
Trauma	26

B

Anaphylaxis

Rash, bronchospasm, hypotension

3

- Increase O_2 to 100%
- Remove suspected trigger(s)
  - If latex is suspected, thoroughly wash area
- Ensure adequate ventilation/oxygenation
- If HYPOtensive, turn off anesthetic agents

Common causative agents:
- Neuromuscular blockers
- Latex
- Chlorhexidine
- IV colloids
- Antibiotics

Purpose	Treatments	Dosage and Administration
To restore intravascular volume	NS or LR	10–30 mL/kg IV/IO, **rapidly**
To restore BP and ↓ mediator release	Epinephrine	1–10 MICROgrams/kg IV/IO, as needed, may need infusion 0.02-0.2 MICROgrams/kg/min
For continued ↓ BP after epinephrine given	Vasopressin	10 MICROunits/kg IV
To ↓ bronchoconstriction	Albuterol (Beta-agonists)	4–10 puffs as needed
To ↓ mediator release	Methylprednisolone	2 mg/kg IV/IO MAX 100 mg
To ↓ histamine-mediated effects	Diphenhydramine	1 mg/kg IV/IO MAX 50 mg
To ↓ effects of histamine	Famotidine or Ranitidine	0.25 mg/kg IV 1 mg/kg IV

- For laboratory confirmation, if needed, send mast cell tryptase level within 2 h of event

Anaphylaxis

Fig. 2. Table of contents (A) and sample page (B) from the Society for Pediatric Anesthesia (SPA) Quality and Safety Committee, PediCrisis Critical Events Checklist. (*From* Society for Pediatric Anesthesia. Critical events checklists. Available at: www.pedsanesthesia.org/critical-events-checklists. Accessed October 12, 2017.)

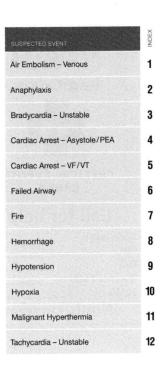

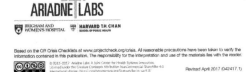

Fig. 3. Table of contents (*A*) and sample page (*B*) from Ariadne Labs, Operating Room Crisis Checklists. (*Courtesy of* Ariadne Labs, Boston, MA. Available at: http://www.projectcheck. org/crisis.html. Accessed October 12, 2017.)

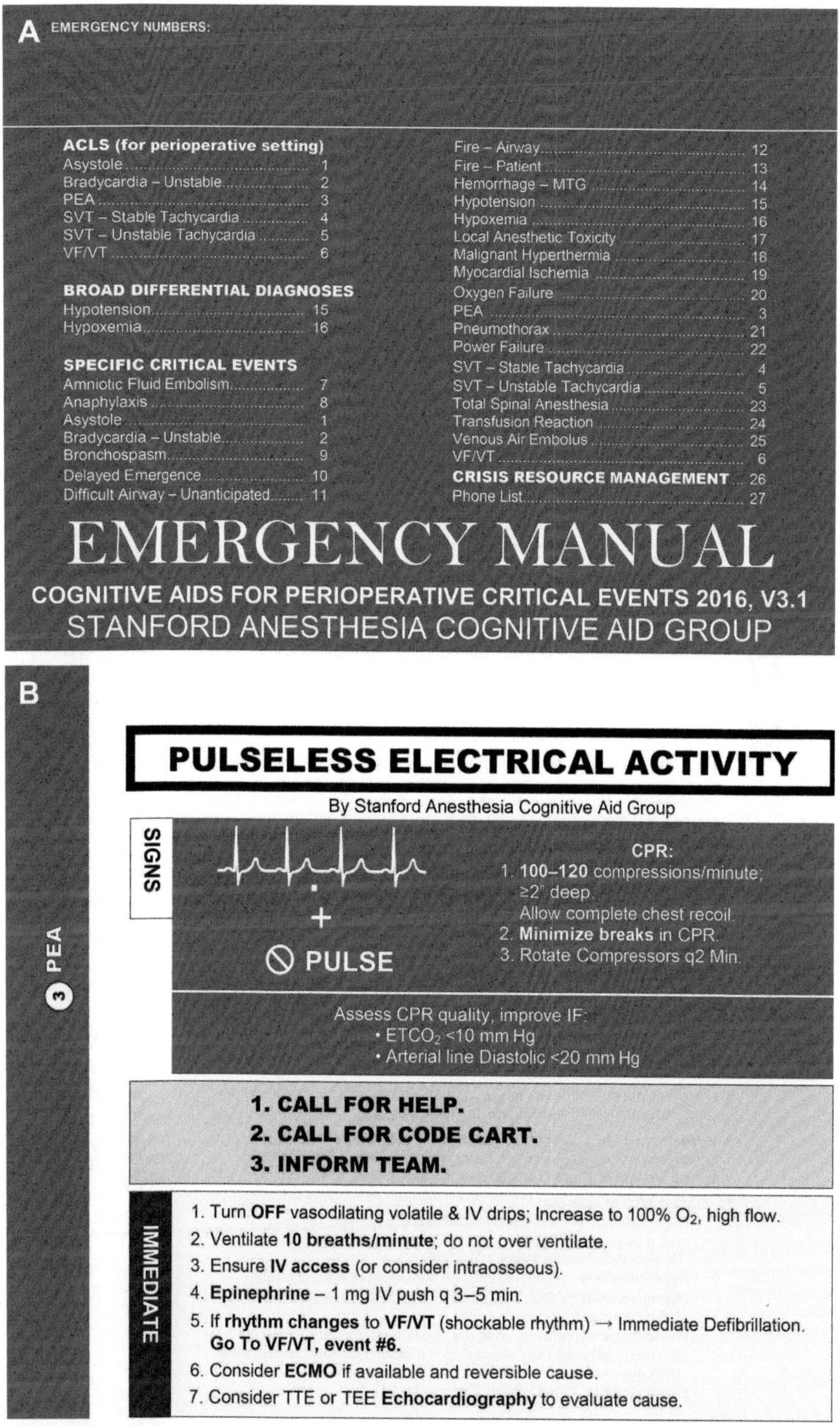

A EMERGENCY NUMBERS:

EMERGENCY MANUAL
COGNITIVE AIDS FOR PERIOPERATIVE CRITICAL EVENTS 2016, V3.1
STANFORD ANESTHESIA COGNITIVE AID GROUP

B

③ PEA

PULSELESS ELECTRICAL ACTIVITY
By Stanford Anesthesia Cognitive Aid Group

SIGNS

⊘ PULSE

CPR:
1. **100–120** compressions/minute; ≥2" deep. Allow complete chest recoil.
2. **Minimize breaks** in CPR.
3. Rotate Compressors q2 Min.

Assess CPR quality, improve IF:
- ETCO$_2$ <10 mm Hg
- Arterial line Diastolic <20 mm Hg

1. CALL FOR HELP.
2. CALL FOR CODE CART.
3. INFORM TEAM.

IMMEDIATE
1. Turn **OFF** vasodilating volatile & IV drips; Increase to 100% O$_2$, high flow.
2. Ventilate **10 breaths/minute**; do not over ventilate.
3. Ensure **IV access** (or consider intraosseous).
4. **Epinephrine** – 1 mg IV push q 3–5 min.
5. If **rhythm changes** to VF/VT (shockable rhythm) → Immediate Defibrillation. **Go To VF/VT, event #6.**
6. Consider **ECMO** if available and reversible cause.
7. Consider TTE or TEE **Echocardiography** to evaluate cause.

Fig. 4. Table of contents (*A*) and sample pages (*B, C*) from Stanford Anesthesia Cognitive Aid Group, Emergency Manual: Cognitive Aids for Perioperative Critical Events, 2016 V3.1. (*Courtesy of* Stanford Anesthesia Cognitive Aid Group. Available at: http://emergencymanual.stanford.edu. Accessed October 12, 2017.)

SECONDARY

Consider common perioperative Ddx:

1. Hemorrhage
2. Anesthetic overdose
3. Septic or other shock states
4. Auto PEEP
5. Anaphylaxis
6. Medication error
7. High spinal
8. Pneumothorax
9. Local anesthetic toxicity
10. Vagal stimulus
11. Pulmonary Embolus

Find and Treat Causes – H's and T's: Expanded on next page.

Go To Next Page□➔

C

PULSELESS ELECTRICAL ACTIVITY *continued*

DETAILS

1. **Hypovolemia:** Give rapid bolus of IV fluid. Check hemoglobin/hematocrit. If anemia or massive hemorrhage, give blood. Consider relative hypovolemia: Auto-PEEP (disconnect circuit); High Spinal; or Shock States (eg anaphylaxis). **Go To relevant event.**

2. **Hypoxemia:** Increase O_2, to 100% high flow. Confirm connections. Check for bilateral breath sounds. Suction ET tube and reconfirm placement. Consider chest X-ray. **Go To Hypoxemia, event #16.**

3. **Tension pneumothorax:** Unilateral breath sounds, possible distended neck veins and deviated trachea (late signs). Perform emergent needle decompression (2nd intercostal space at mid-clavicular line) then chest tube placement. Call for chest x-ray, but do NOT delay treatment. **Go To Pneumothorax, event #21.**

4. **Thrombosis – Coronary:** Consider transesophageal (TEE) or transthoracic (TTE) echocardiography to evaluate ventricle wall motion abnormalities of the ventricles. Consider emergent coronary revascularization. **Go To Myocardial Ischemia, event #19.**

5. **Thrombosis – Pulmonary:** Consider TEE or TTE to evaluate right ventricle. Consider fibrinolytic agents or pulmonary thrombectomy.

6. **Toxins (e.g. infusions):** Consider medication error. Confirm no infusions running and volatile anesthetic off. If local anesthetic toxicity **Go To Local Anesthetic Toxicity, event #17.**

7. **Tamponade – Cardiac:** Consider placing TEE or TTE to rule out tamponade. Treat with pericardiocentesis.

8. **Hypothermia ↓:** Active warming by forced air blanket, warm IV fluid, raise room temperature. Consider cardiopulmonary bypass.

9. **Hyperthermia ↑:** If Malignant Hyperthermia, call for MH Cart. Give Dantrolene immediately: start at 2.5 mg/kg. MH Hotline: (800) 644-9737. **Go To Malignant Hyperthermia, event #18.**

10. **Obtain ABG to rule-out:**
    - **Hyperkalemia ↑:** Give Calcium Chloride 1 g IV; D50 1 Amp IV (25 g Dextrose) + Regular Insulin 10 units IV. Monitor glucose. Sodium Bicarbonate 1 Amp IV (50 mEq).
    - **Hypokalemia ↓:** Controlled infusion of potassium & magnesium.
    - **Hypoglycemia:** If ABG delay, check Fingerstick. Give D50 1 Amp IV (25 g Dextrose). Monitor glucose.
    - **H+ Acidosis:** If profound, consider Sodium Bicarbonate 1 Amp IV (50 mEq). May consider increasing ventilation rate (but can decrease CPR effectiveness so monitor).
    - **Hypocalcemia:** Give Calcium Chloride 1 g IV.

③ PEA

END

Fig. 4. *(continued)*

REFERENCES

1. McEvoy MD, Field LC, Moore HE, et al. The effect of adherence to ACLS protocols on survival of event in the setting of in-hospital cardiac arrest. Resuscitation 2014;85(1):82–7.
2. Harrison TK, Manser T, Howard SK, et al. Use of cognitive aids in a simulated anesthetic crisis. Anesth Analg 2006;103(3):551–6.
3. Neal JM, Hsiung RL, Mulroy MF, et al. ASRA checklist improves trainee performance during a simulated episode of local anesthetic systemic toxicity. Reg Anesth Pain Med 2012;37(1):8–15.
4. Arriaga AF, Bader AM, Wong JM, et al. Simulation-based trial of surgical-crisis checklists. N Engl J Med 2013;368(3):246–53.
5. Emergency Manuals Implementation Collaborative (EMIC). Available at: www.emergencymanuals.org/. Accessed August 22, 2017.
6. Huang J. Implementation of emergency manuals in China. Anesthesia Patient Safety Foundation (APSF) Newsletter 2016;43–5.
7. Dismukes RK, Goldsmith TE, Kochan JA. Effects of acute stress on aircrew performance: literature review and analysis of operational aspects. 2015. Available at: http://human-factors.arc.nasa.gov/publications/NASA_TM_2015_218930-2.pdf. Accessed October 12, 2017.
8. Stiegler MP, Neelankavil JP, Canales C, et al. Cognitive errors detected in anaesthesiology: a literature review and pilot study. Br J Anaesth 2012;108(2):229–35.
9. Gaba DM, Fish KJ, Howard SK, et al. Crisis management in anesthesiology. 2nd edition. Saunders; 2015. 1st edition published by Churchill Livingstone, Inc.
10. Ramirez M, Grantham C. Crisis checklists for the operating room, not with a simulator. J Am Coll Surg 2012;215(2):302–3.
11. Ranganathan P, Phillips JH, Attaallah AF, et al. The use of cognitive aid checklist leading to successful treatment of malignant hyperthermia in an infant undergoing cranioplasty. Anesth Analg 2014;118(6):1387.
12. Goldhaber-Fiebert SN, Pollock J, Howard SK, et al. Emergency manual uses during actual critical events and changes in safety culture from the perspective of anesthesia residents: a pilot study. Anesth Analg 2016;123(3):641–9.
13. Babcock WW. Resuscitation during anesthesia. Anesth Analg 1924;3(6):208–13.
14. Howard SK, Gaba DM, Fish KJ, et al. Anesthesia crisis resource management training: teaching anesthesiologists to handle critical incidents. Aviat Space Environ Med 1992;63(9):763–70.
15. Gaba DM. The future vision of simulation in health care. Qual Saf Health Care 2004;13:I2–10.
16. Clancy CM, Tornberg DN. TeamSTEPPS: assuring optimal teamwork in clinical settings. Am J Med Qual 2007;22(3):214–7.
17. Gawande A. The checklist manifesto: how to get things right. 1st edition. New York: Metropolitan Books; 2010.
18. Schmidt E, Goldhaber-Fiebert SN, Ho LA, et al. Simulation exercises as a patient safety strategy: a systematic review. Ann Intern Med 2013;158(5 Pt 2):426–32.
19. Hepner DL, Arriaga AF, Cooper JB, et al. Operating room crisis checklists and emergency manuals. Anesthesiology 2017;127(2):384–92.
20. Runciman WB, Merry AF. Crises in clinical care: an approach to management. Qual Saf Health Care 2005;14(3):156–63.

21. EMIC Tools. Emergency Manuals Implementation Collaborative (EMIC). Available at: http://www.emergencymanuals.org/free-tools.html. Accessed August 22, 2017.

22. Hales BM, Pronovost PJ. The checklist: a tool for error management and performance improvement. J Crit Care 2006;21(3):231–5.

23. Haynes AB, Weiser TG, Berry WR, et al. A surgical safety checklist to reduce morbidity and mortality in a global population. N Engl J Med 2009;360(5):491–9.

24. Gaba DM, Pierce EC Jr. Patient safety memorial lecture: competence and teamwork are not enough: the value of cognitive aids. In: American Society of Anesthesiologists Annual Meeting; 2014. Available at: http://www.asahq.org/sitecore/content/Annual-Meeting/Education/Featured-Lectures/Ellison-Pierce-Memorial-Lecture.aspx. Accessed August 22, 2017.

25. Goldhaber-Fiebert SN, Howard SK. Implementing emergency manuals: can cognitive aids help translate best practices for patient care during acute events? Anesth Analg 2013;117(5):1149–61.

26. Damschroder LJ, Aron DC, Keith RE, et al. Fostering implementation of health services research findings into practice: a consolidated framework for advancing implementation science. Implement Sci 2009;4:50.

27. Powell BJ, Waltz TJ, Chinman MJ, et al. A refined compilation of implementation strategies: results from the Expert Recommendations for Implementing Change (ERIC) project. Implement Sci 2015;10:21.

28. Implementing and using emergency manuals and checklists to improve patient safety: Anesthesia Patient Safety Foundation (APSF) Expert's Conference. Phoenix, AZ; September 9, 2015.

29. Burden AR, Carr ZJ, Staman GW, et al. Does every code need a "reader?" improvement of rare event management with a cognitive aid "reader" during a simulated emergency: a pilot study. Simul Healthc 2012;7(1):1–9.

30. Bould MD, Hayter MA, Campbell DM, et al. Cognitive aid for neonatal resuscitation: a prospective single-blinded randomized controlled trial. Br J Anaesth 2009; 103(4):570–5.

31. Marshall S. The use of cognitive aids during emergencies in anesthesia: a review of the literature. Anesth Analg 2013;117(5):1162–71.

32. Marshall SD, Mehra R. The effects of a displayed cognitive aid on non-technical skills in a simulated "can't intubate, can't oxygenate" crisis. Anaesthesia 2014; 69(7):669–77.

33. Marshall SD, Sanderson P, McIntosh CA, et al. The effect of two cognitive aid designs on team functioning during intra-operative anaphylaxis emergencies: a multi-centre simulation study. Anaesthesia 2016;71(4):389–404.

34. Watkins SC, Anders S, Clebone A, et al. Paper or plastic? Simulation based evaluation of two versions of a cognitive aid for managing pediatric peri-operative critical events by anesthesia trainees: evaluation of the society for pediatric anesthesia emergency checklist. J Clin Monit Comput 2016;30(3):275–83.

35. Watkins SC, Anders S, Clebone A, et al. Mode of information delivery does not effect anesthesia trainee performance during simulated perioperative pediatric critical events: a trial of paper versus electronic cognitive aids. Simul Healthc 2016;11(6):385.

36. Neily J, DeRosier JM, Mills PD, et al. Awareness and use of a cognitive aid for anesthesiology. Jt Comm J Qual Patient Saf 2007;33(8):502–11.

37. Ariadne Labs. OR crisis checklists. www.projectcheck.org/crisis.html. Accessed August 22, 2017.

38. Stanford Anesthesia Cognitive Aid Group (SACAG). Stanford emergency manual: cognitive aids for perioperative critical events. Stanford emergency manual: cognitive aids for perioperative critical events. Available at: http://emergencymanual.stanford.edu. Accessed October 12, 2017.
39. Society for Pediatric Anesthesia. Pediatric critical events checklists. Available at: http://www.pedsanesthesia.org/critical-events-checklists/. Accessed August 22, 2017.
40. Goldhaber-Fiebert SN, Lei V, Nandagopal K, et al. Emergency manual implementation: can brief simulation-based OR staff trainings increase familiarity and planned clinical use? Jt Comm J Qual Patient Saf 2015;41(5):212–7.
41. Goldhaber-Fiebert SN, Lei V, Jackson ML, et al. Simulation-based team training: crisis resource management and the use of emergency manuals in the OR. MedEDPORTAL Publications. 2014: Available at: https://www.mededportal.org/publication/9992. Accessed October 12, 2017.
42. Goldhaber-Fiebert SN. Why and how to implement emergency manuals. 2013. Available at: https://www.youtube.com/watch?v=shc1BBzslyI. Accessed October 12, 2017.
43. Goldhaber-Fiebert SN, Lei V, Bereknyei Merrell S, et al. Perioperative emergency manuals in clinical clerkships: curricula on "why, how, and when to use" for teaching medical students. MedEdPORTAL Publications. 2015: Available at: https://www.mededportal.org/publication/10056. Accessed October 12, 2017.
44. Ariadne Labs. OR crisis checklists. OR crisis checklists training videos. Available at: https://youtu.be/iaHiSYR11u0. Accessed August 22, 2017.
45. Bosk CL, Dixon-Woods M, Goeschel CA, et al. Reality check for checklists. Lancet 2009;374(9688):444–5.
46. Batalden P. Making improvement interventions happen—the work before the work: four leaders speak. BMJ Qual Saf 2014;23(1):4–7.
47. Dixon-Woods M, Bosk CL, Aveling EL, et al. Explaining Michigan: developing an ex post theory of a quality improvement program. Milbank Q 2011;89(2):167–205.
48. Dixon-Woods M, Leslie M, Tarrant C, et al. Explaining matching Michigan: an ethnographic study of a patient safety program. Implement Sci 2013;8:70.
49. Catchpole K, Russ S. The problem with checklists. BMJ Qual Saf 2015;24(9):545–9.
50. Russ SJ, Sevdalis N, Moorthy K, et al. A qualitative evaluation of the barriers and facilitators toward implementation of the WHO surgical safety checklist across hospitals in England: lessons from the "surgical checklist implementation project". Ann Surg 2015;261(1):81–91.
51. Dixon-Woods M, Leslie M, Bion J, et al. What counts? An ethnographic study of infection data reported to a patient safety program. Milbank Q 2012;90(3):548–91.
52. Macrae C, Draycott T. Delivering high reliability in maternity care: in situ simulation as a source of organisational resilience. Saf Sci 2016. https://doi.org/10.1016/j.ssci.2016.10.019.
53. Draycott T, Sagar R, Hogg S. The role of insurers in maternity safety. Best Pract Res Clin Obstet Gynaecol 2015;29(8):1126–31.
54. Denis JL, Hébert Y, Langley A, et al. Explaining diffusion patterns for complex health care innovations. Health Care Manage Rev 2002;27(3):60.
55. Clay-Williams R, Colligan L. Back to basics: checklists in aviation and healthcare. BMJ Qual Saf 2015;24(7):428–31.

56. Schulman PR. The negotiated order of organizational reliability. Adm Soc 1993; 25(3):353–72.
57. Macrae C. Close calls: managing risk and resilience in airline flight safety. Palgrave Macmillan; 2014.
58. Dixon-Woods M, McNicol S, Martin G. Ten challenges in improving quality in healthcare: lessons from the Health Foundation's programme evaluations and relevant literature. BMJ Qual Saf 2012;21(10):876–84.

Use of Simulation in Performance Improvement

Amanda Burden, MD*, Erin White Pukenas, MD

KEYWORDS

- Performance improvement • Patient safety • Simulation education • Leadership
- Feedback • Crisis resource management • Team management • Communication

KEY POINTS

- Despite increased attention and focus, human error and system failures continue to lead to preventable patient care errors.
- Simulation has proven to be an effective educational tool to address medical technical skills, communication skills, and teamwork skills.
- Simulation has recently been used as part of performance improvement strategies for attending physicians and teams.

Despite ongoing attention and efforts to improve patient safety, medical errors persist. In the United States in 1999, the Institute of Medicine (now the National Academy of Medicine) estimated that between 44,000 and 98,000 people die yearly because of medical errors.[1] Recent studies estimate that the true number of premature deaths due to preventable patient harm may be much larger, suggesting that more than 400,000 such deaths occur each year.[2] Although these deaths are at times the result of inadequate medical knowledge and skill, they commonly occur because of inadequate communication and poor management of situation and team dynamics.[1–4] Overcoming these individual and team failures requires dedicated efforts aimed at improving performance and practice.[5–7] Simulation represents one such effort that has found usefulness in training and in maintaining individual and team performance.

A BRIEF HISTORY OF PERFORMANCE IMPROVEMENT

Early performance improvement efforts can be traced as far back as ancient Greece in the work of Hippocrates and Asclepius.[8] In more recent times, Ignaz Semmelweis[9] is recognized as one of the first physicians to demonstrate significant improvement in patient outcomes after instituting a clinical practice change. While reflecting on the

Disclosure Statement: Both authors have nothing to disclose.
Cooper Medical School of Rowan University, 401 South Broadway Camden, NJ 08103, USA
* Corresponding author.
E-mail address: burdena@rowan.edu

Anesthesiology Clin 36 (2018) 63–74
https://doi.org/10.1016/j.anclin.2017.10.001
1932-2275/18/© 2017 Elsevier Inc. All rights reserved.

practice habits of his colleagues and medical students in the 1840s, Semmelweis noted the lack of hand sanitization after autopsy performance. These same physicians and medical students would then examine pregnant women after merely wiping their hands on their dirty autopsy aprons. Semmelweis's efforts to promote handwashing among his colleagues and medical students resulted in an 80% reduction in maternal deaths.[9]

In the 1910s, surgeon Ernest Codman's "End Result Idea" was introduced in the United States.[10] Codman advocated tracking patient outcomes to determine whether treatment was successful and why treatments failed. His system to prevent future failures mirrored the well-known plan-do-study-act (PDSA) cycles of today. Since then, performance improvement has evolved into an applied science with a more scientifically rigorous approach to learning.[11] A variety of educational strategies have been introduced to address individual and team performance improvement. This article focuses on the use of simulation education as a strategy to improve medical practice, reduce medical errors, and improve patient safety.

SIMULATION DEFINED

Simulation "is a technique to replace or amplify real-patient experiences with guided experiences, artificially contrived, that evokes or replicates substantial aspects of the real world in a fully interactive manner."[12] Simulation provides an educational opportunity that is immersive and experiential. Simulation can involve many forms, including simulated and virtual patients, static and interactive mannequin simulators, task trainers, screen-based (computer) simulations, and computer games. Simulation has the potential to recreate rarely experienced scenarios, allowing professionals to work in challenging situations with the opportunity to carefully replay or examine their actions.[13] Best practice in simulation education indicates that certain key features and conditions must accompany simulation-based education to allow for optimal learning outcomes. These include simulator validity, feedback, deliberate and repetitive practice, curriculum integration, ranges of difficulty, multiple learning strategies, a controlled environment, individualized learning, clinical variation, and defining outcomes (**Box 1**).[14] When

---

Box 1
Features of simulation that contribute to effective learning

Feedback: MOST important, provides opportunity for reflection and practice improvement

Repetitive practice with the use of feedback to allow for deliberate practice

Varying degrees of difficulty needed to allow the learner to progress

Multiple learning strategies should be used

Clinical variation should be appropriate and relevant to participants' practice

Faculty should be able to control the environment

Opportunities for individualized learning should exist

Programs and courses should have defined outcomes and benchmarks

The simulated environment should be realistic

Simulation program should be integrated into a curriculum

Data from Issenberg SB, McGaghie WC, Petrusa ER, et al. Features and uses of high-fidelity medical simulations that lead to effective learning: a BEME systematic review. Med Teach 2005;27(1):10–28.

executed according to these principles, simulation is a powerful learning tool that health care professionals can use to achieve higher levels of competence and safer care.[4,12,15,16]

SIMULATION EDUCATION: ANESTHESIOLOGISTS AT THE FOREFRONT

Anesthesiologists have led the creation and expansion of simulation-based medical education beginning in the early twentieth century. Interest in this educational methodology has expanded greatly during the past decade. More medical schools and hospitals are building simulation programs, and credentialing bodies are beginning to require the addition of simulation to both educational and certification processes. The leadership of anesthesiologists in simulation continues to be a critical force in advancing the science of performance improvement (**Table 1**).

The earliest record of the use of simulation to educate physicians can be traced to the "anatomy laboratory" that was created by anesthesiologist John Lundy.[17] Lundy, head of anesthesia for the Mayo Clinic in the 1920s, first developed a program to educate surgical fellows in anatomy, hoping to both improve their performance of regional anesthesia and as part of an effort to interest them and other physicians in the emerging field of anesthesiology. He created the anatomy laboratory, which consisted of cadavers, so the fellows would be able to practice procedures. Initially used by surgical residents, it ultimately became a multidisciplinary laboratory.[18,19]

Lundy[18,19] observed that surgical fellows who studied in his laboratory before assisting with patients in the operating room (OR) better understood the anatomy and regional anesthesia techniques on live patients than those who had not. Lundy[18,19] developed a simulation program that recreated the OR environment so residents could practice under OR-like conditions. This allowed the surgical fellows to practice procedures, learn anatomy, and receive feedback about their performance, all of which remain extremely valuable features of simulation today.

Inspired by research into medical error, patient safety, and human factors by scientist Jeffrey Cooper and colleagues[3,15] in the 1970s, anesthesiologists have led health care performance improvement efforts for several decades. The research by Cooper and colleagues[3,15] was among the influences leading to the formation of the Anesthesia Patient Safety Foundation (APSF), which was established to continually

Table 1
Anesthesiology leaders in simulation

Date	Scientist	Contribution
1920s	Lundy	Created laboratory environment to teach physicians practice of regional techniques and to deal with patient challenges in operating room environment
1960s	Safar, Lund	Created process for CPR and forced ventilation, CPR mannequin
1960s	Denson	Created Sim One, first physiologically realistic mannequin
1970s	Cooper	Identified human factors errors in anesthesia incidents, work led to founding of APSF
1980s	Gaba	Created Anesthesia Crisis Resource Management; created simulator and realistic simulated environment
1980s	Good, Gravenstein	Created computerized simulator: Gainesville Anesthesia Simulator

Abbreviations: APSF, Anesthesia Patient Safety Foundation; CPR, cardiopulmonary resuscitation.
   Data from Cooper JB, Taqueti VR. A brief history of the development of mannequin simulators for clinical education and training. Qual Saf Health Care 2004;13(suppl 1):i11–8.

improve the safety of patients during anesthesia care by encouraging and conducting research and education in safety.[4,20]

With funding from APSF, anesthesiologist David Gaba and colleagues[16,21,22] at Stanford and the Veterans Affairs Palo Alto Health Care System developed the prototype of a mannequin simulator. This new mannequin could exhibit vital signs that could be manipulated to simulate critical events. It was housed in a real OR and was surrounded by functional equipment, which created a highly realistic simulation environment to investigate human performance.[16,21,22] While performing cardiopulmonary bypass experiments involving animals, Gaba and colleagues[16,21] investigated decision making during patient emergencies. They adapted "crew resource management," an approach to team training used in aviation, to the anesthesia environment, and called it Anesthesia Crisis Resource Management (ACRM).[16,21] The hallmarks of ACRM include leadership, teamwork, distribution of workload, communication, use of all available information and resources, and constant reevaluation of the clinical situation. Gaba and colleagues[16,21] used simulation to present and teach ACRM to anesthesiologists and explored clinicians' actions and decision making in dynamic environments.

PRINCIPLES OF SIMULATION EDUCATION

Simulation may be used by health care professionals to improve performance in a variety of areas. Simulation can be used to learn, improve, and enhance performance of technical procedures.[23] Simulated or standardized patients are also used to teach and assess clinical skills.[24] Simulation also has been used to allow teams to train so they may improve function in tension-filled complex situations.[25] Benefits of simulation education include the ability to standardize and repeat content, the opportunity for interactive learning in a clinical setting without patient risk, and the ability to specifically design clinical experiences.[26]

Simulation to educate health care practitioners has been shown to be effective in transferring knowledge to both trainees and practicing health care professionals. Several studies have documented transfer of training to patient care settings.[27–33] Barsuk and colleagues[27–29] studied internal medicine residents and showed that trainees who have mastered central venous catheter insertion in a simulation laboratory have significantly fewer procedural complications (eg, needle passes) in an intensive care unit (ICU) than residents who are not simulation-trained. In obstetrics, Draycott and colleagues[31,34] published extensive research demonstrating improved neonatal outcomes of births complicated by shoulder dystocia after the implementation of simulation-based training. Within the surgical domain, several studies have demonstrated that simulator-trained individuals are faster, more accurate, and commit fewer errors during their first real case.[35,36]

There are 3 key principles that should be followed to promote the effective use of simulation: encouraging deliberate practice (DP), teaching and assessing nontechnical skills, and replicating reality.

Encouraging Deliberate Practice

A critical aspect of simulation education is to provide learners with an opportunity for DP.[37] DP involves consistent educational interventions aimed at skill acquisition, maintenance, and continual improvement.[5,37] The power of DP has been demonstrated in many professional domains, including sports, commerce, performing arts, science, and writing.[5] Research shows that DP is a much more powerful predictor of professional accomplishment than experience or academic aptitude.[5,37] DP is especially useful for education surrounding technical skills, but also has been used to allow learners to reflect on and improve their performance of nontechnical skills (eg, communication, teamwork, decision making).[12,38–40] Using simulation to teach these skills allows students to make mistakes in a safe environment, learn from those mistakes, and achieve proficiency.[12,38] Simulation education with DP has demonstrated effectiveness at improving skills for a variety of procedures and processes (eg, central lines, lumbar puncture, intubations, and patient handoffs).[27–29,41–44]

Teaching and Assessing Nontechnical Skills

Bringing members of the health care team together in a simulated environment enables team training to explore communication, decision-making, judgment, and leadership skills.[4,15,39] Although this approach uses many resources and significant time, it has been shown to be a feasible and instructive technique for OR, ICU, and labor and delivery teams in the simulation laboratory or in the clinical environment itself.[30,34,45] A few studies report improved individual and team response in acute and ambulatory care settings following a team simulation session.[30,31,39,46] Crisis scenarios can be played out with extensive debriefing performed on an individual and team basis.

The focus on teamwork in simulation reflects a growing appreciation of the need for health care personnel to work as part of a collaborative team to affect optimal patient care, and that this should be a focus for educational efforts throughout medical education and training.[1,4,12,33] The Institute of Medicine recommends interprofessional health care education as a critical patient safety strategy.[1] Improving teamwork to improve safety has been widely applied in a variety of high-risk industries, most notably with the use of Crew Resource Management (CRM) in the airline industry. Similar CRM initiatives have been used to improve patient safety. A recent collaboration between the Agency for Healthcare Research and Quality (AHRQ) and the US Department of Defense resulted in the development of the TeamSTEPPS simulation-based curriculum to improve patient safety through enhanced communication and other teamwork skills.[47] One of the core competency areas of TeamSTEPPS is team leadership, which includes the ability to direct and coordinate activities of team members, assess team performance, assign tasks, develop team knowledge and skills, motivate team members, plan and organize, and establish a positive team atmosphere.[47]

Replicating Reality

Another important aspect of simulation-based training is its ability to replicate the real environment. Wayne and colleagues[46] demonstrated that Advanced Cardiac Life Support skills acquired by internal medicine residents in a simulation laboratory do not decay at 6 and 14 months after training. Bruppacher and colleagues[48] performed a study comparing traditional education using an interactive lecture versus simulation education to teach anesthesiology residents cardiopulmonary bypass (CPB) weaning. Senior trainees, who were all inexperienced in CPB weaning, received a focused training session via a high-fidelity simulation or an interactive lecture. The simulation group scored significantly higher than the seminar group during a blinded clinical observation of CPB weaning on 2 different testing occasions. Transfer of both technical and nontechnical skills to the clinical setting from simulation education was noted.[48]

SIMULATION AND CONTINUING EDUCATION FOR PHYSICIAN ANESTHESIOLOGISTS

In 2004, the American Society of Anesthesiologists (ASA) appointed a Workgroup on Simulation Education that intended to identify programs appropriate for continuing medical education for attending physician anesthesiologists. In 2006, the workgroup drafted a White Paper, "ASA Approval of Anesthesiology Simulation Programs." Concurrently, the workgroup conducted a survey of ASA members, which revealed that most (81%) of the 1350 ASA member respondents had an interest in simulation-based continuing medical education (CME), with a similar percentage (77%) indicating they felt simulation-based CME offered benefits superior to those offered by traditional, lecture-based CME. ASA members identified that features of simulation-based training that were most meaningful were a realistic mannequin (77%), a high instructor-to-student ratio (76%), and a realistic simulation of the environment (69%). Videotaping of performance (51%) and multidisciplinary training (50%) were less frequently identified as important elements of simulation-based CME. Additionally, 71% sought an assessment of their performance, intending to use this educational method to improve their practice.[49] Also in 2006, the ASA Committee on Simulation Education was formed to foster access to high-quality simulation-based education for ASA members. To accomplish this mission, the committee developed a list of educational, faculty development, and program criteria required to receive ASA endorsement and established the Simulation Education Network[49,50] (**Table 2**). Charged by the American Board of Anesthesiology (ABA) in 2010, the committee developed simulation courses aimed at allowing physician anesthesiologists to reflect on and improve their performance. Simulation became an approved component of the Part 4 Maintenance of Certification in Anesthesiology (MOCA) requirement in 2010.[49,51]

SIMULATION AND THE AMERICAN BOARD OF ANESTHESIOLOGY

The ABA initially proposed simulation as a mechanism for Part 4 of MOCA, the practice improvement section, in January 2010.[49,51] Simulation courses were chosen for these programs for several reasons:

Table 2
Essential elements for American Society of Anesthesiologists Simulation Education Network

Program overview	Programs should detail their mission statement and overall program goals
Educational programs	Endorsed programs must have robust educational offerings for anesthesiology students, residents, and attending physicians
Scenario	Scenario must be appropriate and relevant for attending physician–level education
Curriculum development	Programs must have a standard process for developing courses and curricula
Instructor and faculty development	Programs must have ongoing faculty development programs for instructors
Leadership	Program director must have appropriate education in use of simulation, institutional support, and time to dedicate to program
Facility and equipment	Infrastructure must be appropriate to support continuing medical education offerings
Policies and procedures	Program must address issues of confidentiality and performance anxiety, and must continually evaluate and seek to improve its offerings

Data from Steadman RH. The American Society of Anesthesiologists' national endorsement program for simulation centers. J Crit Care 2008;23(2):203–6.

1. Simulation has demonstrated the ability to engage participants and stimulate reflection and behavior change,[12,15] which made it likely that participants would self-assess and identify gaps in their practice.
2. Simulation can allow participants to practice managing critical events that rarely occur.
3. Anesthesiologists can view their performance on video and reflect on opportunities for improvement.[49,51]

The simulation courses consist of a 1-day simulation course at one of the ASA-endorsed simulation centers. The MOCA Simulation Courses address both medical and technical skills required to manage acute perioperative challenges, as well as the nontechnical skills of team management and decision making. The sessions are debriefed and participants are able to reflect on their performances after each scenario. This allows them to identify areas in their practice that they would like to improve. The practice improvements are submitted to the ASA; the participants then attempt to implement these changes and report back about their success and what barriers they faced. MOCA simulation is not a test, but is a personal practice assessment and improvement activity.[49,51–53]

The initial experience with the MOCA simulation activity has been very positive. In follow-up surveys, 95% of participants reported that they would recommend simulation to their colleagues, and 98% felt the course was relevant to their practice. Course participants have identified relevance as the most important element of the program. Follow-up surveys identified that 95% of participants had successfully completed changes in their practice based on what they identified during the course.[51]

For many of the participants, these courses generated impressive and impactful improvements. The follow-up results for more than 1800 self-identified practice improvement plans were reviewed; participants completed many compelling and impactful plans. The participants often overcame barriers and exceeded the scope of their original plans. Examples include plans demonstrating direct benefits for patients related to improving teamwork and communication skills. Others included widespread dissemination of management guidelines, such as emergency manuals, across departments and hospital networks. Interprofessional collaboration was remarkable in many instances. Additionally, a participant reported that he used intraosseous insertion techniques he learned during a MOCA simulation course to save a patient's life.[53,54]

Recently, AHRQ funded a study conducted by an interdisciplinary team from 12 academic institutions that sought to determine whether standardized mannequin-based simulation can reliably characterize how experienced physicians would manage medical emergencies.[55] Participants were video recorded, allowing independent experts to rate the technical and behavioral performance of the clinicians. Although the study found that approximately 80% of critical actions were performed and three-quarters of the overall performances were rated as average or better on the rating scales, opportunities to improve were identified, thus indicating ways to make perioperative care even safer. Important findings identified that one of the simplest actions, calling for help, proved to be quite effective, as the arrival of a second experienced physician nearly always improved care. Although the study methods were not able to determine competence, ability, or skill of individual clinicians, the scenarios were able to investigate the spectrum of performance seen in complex simulations of well-known crisis events. Opportunities for practice improvement included escalating therapy when the initial response was ineffective, engaging other team members (especially when some action by them is required), and following evidence-based guidelines in some cases.[55]

SIMULATION AND MEDICAL MALPRACTICE

Medical malpractice insurance companies have identified opportunities to use simulation to spur performance improvement. The Risk Management Foundation of the Harvard Medical Institutions (CRICO) is a patient safety and medical malpractice company that is owned by and serves the Harvard medical community. In 2001, the CRICO Risk Management Foundation began offering insurance premium incentives for anesthesiologists who participated in simulation-based crisis resource management courses.[56,57] After several years of sponsoring these simulation courses, CRICO members analyzed malpractice claims and concluded that the program had reduced both the number and cost of malpractice claims. The company subsequently increased the value of the premium incentives for anesthesiologists who participated in these courses. The benefit was large enough that CRICO also worked with the simulation experts to create similar programs in other specialties and a team training program for OR teams.[56,57] Other malpractice insurance companies have now made this type of training a component of a group of patient safety provisions that can lead to a reduction in premiums.[57–59]

SIMULATION AND FUTURE RESEARCH

The AHRQ, APSF, Foundation for Education and Research in Anesthesia, and many other specialty societies have allocated funds for simulation research. Furthermore, consensus meetings with simulation experts have generated many questions for collaborative research.[60] As interest in simulation has grown, considerable resources have been dedicated to simulation-based training centers. In addition to the ASA and ABA efforts described earlier, other clinical specialty societies also have established standing committees to endorse simulation education programs. The American College of Surgeons (ACS) created a consortium of ACS-accredited Education Institutes. These programs offer "global opportunities for collaboration, research, and access to resources" designed to enhance patient safety through simulation. A full description of their application process and programs can be found on the ACS Web site.[61] The interprofessional Society for Simulation in Healthcare, whose mission is to "facilitate excellence in health care education, practice, and research through simulation," also offers accreditation as a quality control for simulation training and research.[62]

SUMMARY

The public demands that physicians maintain and improve their skills, but traditional CME activities are not frequently associated with a change in practice.[63–65] Rarely have other CME programs or educational methodologies been able to demonstrate improvement in practice and transfer from learning to clinical environments.[63–66]

Anesthesiologists have demonstrated a long tradition of identifying errors or deficiencies in practice and establishing training programs to improve performance. Anesthesiologists were among the first to advocate for the safety of patients, even in the face of opposition and long before it was popular. Anesthesiologists have contributed many innovative therapies to the medical community and to patient care that are used each day to make patient care safer. Simulation is one of these many tools.

REFERENCES

1. Kohn LT, Corrigan J, Donaldson MS. To err is human: building a safer health system. Washington, DC: National Academies Press; 1999.

2. James JT. A new, evidence-based estimate of patient harms associated with hospital care. J Patient Saf 2013;9(3):122–8.
3. Cooper JB, Newbower RS, Long CD, et al. Preventable anesthesia mishaps: a study of human factors. Anesthesiology 1978;49(6):399–406.
4. Gaba DM, Fish KJ, Howard SK, et al. Crisis management in anesthesiology. 2nd edition. Philadelphia: Elsevier; 2014.
5. Ericsson KA. Deliberate practice and the acquisition and maintenance of expert performance in medicine and related domains. Acad Med 2004;79(10 suppl): S70–81.
6. Smith KK, Gilcreast D, Pierce K. Evaluation of staff's retention of ACLS and BLS skills. Resuscitation 2008;78:59–65.
7. Weaver SJ, Lubomksi LH, Wilson RF, et al. Promoting a culture of safety as a patient safety strategy: a systematic review. Ann Intern Med 2013;158(5 pt 2): 369–74.
8. Fabre J. Hip, hip, Hippocrates: extracts from the Hippocratic doctor. BMJ 1997; 315(7123):1669–70.
9. Semmelweis IP. The cause, concept and prophylaxis of childhood fever 1861.
10. Donabedian A. The end results of health care: Dr. Ernest Codman's contribution to quality assessment and beyond. Milbank Q 1989;67:233–56.
11. Marshall M, Pronovost M, Dixon-Woods M. Promotion of improvement as a science. Lancet 2013;381:419–21.
12. Gaba DM. The future vision of simulation in health care. Qual Saf Health Care 2004;13(suppl 1):i2–10.
13. Agency for Healthcare Research and Quality. Medical errors: the scope of the problem. Rockville (MD): Agency for Healthcare Research and Quality; 2009. Ref Type: Pamphlet.
14. Issenberg SB, McGaghie WC, Petrusa ER, et al. Features and uses of high fidelity medical simulations that lead to effective learning: a BEME systematic review. Med Teach 2005;27(1):10–28.
15. Cooper JB, Taqueti VR. A brief history of the development of mannequin simulators for clinical education and training. Qual Saf Health Care 2004;13(suppl 1): i11–8.
16. Gaba DM, Howard SK, Fish K, et al. Simulation-based training in anesthesia crisis resource management (ACRM): a decade of experience. Simulation Gaming 2001;32(2):175–93.
17. Lundy JS. Anatomy Service Report, February 14, 1929. In the Collected Papers of John S. Lundy, Mayo Foundation Archive, Rochester, Minn; 1929.
18. Ellis TA 2nd, Bacon DR. The anatomy laboratory: a concept ahead of its time. Mayo Clin Proc 2003;78(2):250–1.
19. Lundy JS. Twenty-one months' experience in operating a dissecting room under the Mayo Foundation. In the Collected Papers of John S. Lundy, Mayo Foundation Archive, Rochester, Minn; July 12, 1927.
20. Anesthesia Patient Safety Foundation. Available at: www.apsf.org. Accessed July 2, 2017.
21. Howard SK, Gaba DM, Fish KJ, et al. Anesthesia crisis resource management training: teaching anesthesiologists to handle critical incidents. Aviat Space Environ Med 1992;63(9):763–70.
22. Holzman RS, Cooper JB, Gaba DM, et al. Anesthesia crisis resource management: real-life simulation training in operating room crises. J Clin Anesth 1995; 7(8):675–87.

23. McGaghie WC, Issenberg SB, Cohen ME, et al. Does simulation-based medical education with deliberate practice yield better results than traditional clinical education? A meta-analytic comparative review of the evidence. Acad Med 2011; 86(6):706.

24. Harden RM, Gleeson FA. Assessment of clinical competence using an objective structured clinical examination (OSCE). Med Educ 1979;13:41–54.

25. Salas E, DiazGranados D, Klein C, et al. Does team training improve team performance? A meta-analysis. Hum Factors 2008;50:903–33.

26. Gordon JA, Wilkerson WM, Shaffer DW, et al. "Practicing" medicine without risk: Students' and educators' responses to high-fidelity patient simulation. Acad Med 2001;76:469–72.

27. Barsuk JH, McGaghie WC, Cohen ER, et al. Simulation-based mastery learning reduces complications during central venous catheter insertion in a medical intensive care unit. Crit Care Med 2009;37:2697–701.

28. Cohen ER, Feinglass J, Barsuk JH, et al. Cost savings from reduced catheter-related bloodstream infection after simulation-based education for residents in a medical intensive care unit. Simul Healthc 2010;5:98–102.

29. Burden AR, Torjman MC, Dy GE, et al. Prevention of central venous catheter-related bloodstream infections: is it time to add simulation training to the prevention bundle? J Clin Anesth 2012;24(7):555–60.

30. Hunt EA, Heine M, Hohenhaus SM, et al. Simulated pediatric trauma team management: assessment of an educational intervention. Pediatr Emerg Care 2007; 23:796–804.

31. Draycott TJ, Crofts JF, Ash JP, et al. Improving neonatal outcome through practical shoulder dystocia training. Obstet Gynecol 2008;112:14–20.

32. Andreatta P, Saxton E, Thompson M, et al. Simulation-based mock codes significantly correlate with improved pediatric patient cardiopulmonary arrest survival rates. Pediatr Crit Care Med 2011;12(1):33–8.

33. Morey JC, Simon R, Jay GD, et al. Error reduction and performance improvement in the emergency department through formal teamwork training: evaluation results of the MedTeams project. Health Serv Res 2002;37:1553–81.

34. Draycott T, Sibanda T, Owen L, et al. Does training in obstetric emergencies improve neonatal outcome? BJOG 2006;113:177–82.

35. Seymour NE, Gallagher AG, Roman SA, et al. Virtual reality training improves operating room performance: results of a randomized, double-blinded study. Ann Surg 2002;236(4):458.

36. Gallagher AG, Ritter EM, Champion H, et al. Virtual reality simulation for the operating room: proficiency-based training as a paradigm shift in surgical skills training. Ann Surg 2005;241(2):364.

37. Ericsson KA. Deliberate practice and acquisition of expert performance: a general overview. Acad Emerg Med 2008;15(11):988–94.

38. Steadman RH, Huang YM. Simulation for quality assurance in training, credentialing and maintenance of certification. Best Pract Res Clin Anaesthesiol 2012; 26(1):3–15.

39. Burden AR, Pukenas EW, Deal ER, et al. Using simulation education with deliberate practice to teach leadership and resource management skills to senior resident code leaders. J Grad Med Education 2014;6(3):463–9.

40. Wayne DB, Butter J, Siddall VJ, et al. Simulation-based training of internal medicine residents in advanced cardiac life support protocols: a randomized trial. Teach Learn Med 2005;17:202–8.

41. Issenberg SB, McGaghie WC, Gordon DL, et al. Effectiveness of a cardiology review course for internal medicine residents using simulation technology and deliberate practice. Teach Learn Med 2002;14:223–8.
42. Wayne DB, Didwania A, Feinglass J, et al. Simulation-based education improves quality of care during cardiac arrest team responses at an academic teaching hospital. Chest 2008;133:56–61.
43. Barsuk JH, McGaghie WC, Cohen ER, et al. Use of simulation-based mastery learning to improve the quality of central venous catheter placement in a medical intensive care unit. J Hosp Med 2009;4:397–403.
44. Pukenas EW, Dodson G, Deal ER, et al. Simulation-based education with deliberate practice may improve intraoperative handoff skills: a pilot study. J Clin Anesth 2014;26(7):530–8.
45. Moorthy K, Munz Y, Adams S, et al. A human factors analysis of technical and team skills among surgical trainees during procedural simulations in a simulated operating theatre. Ann Surg 2005;242:631–9.
46. Wayne DB, Siddall VJ, Butter J, et al. A longitudinal study of internal medicine residents' retention of advanced cardiac life support skills. Acad Med 2006; 81(10 Suppl):S9–12.
47. Clancy CM, Tornberg DN. TeamSTEPPS: assuring optimal teamwork in clinical settings. Am J Med Qual 2007;22:214–7.
48. Bruppacher HR, Alam SK, LeBlanc VR, et al. Simulation-based training improves physicians' performance in patient care in high-stakes clinical setting of cardiac surgery. Anesthesiology 2010;112(4):985–92.
49. Steadman RH, Berry AJ, Coursin DB, et al. Simulation and MOCA®: ASA and ABA perspective, after the first three years. ASA Newsl 2013;77(8):30–2.
50. Steadman RH. The American Society of Anesthesiologists' national endorsement program for simulation centers. J Crit Care 2008;23(2):203–6.
51. McIvor W, Burden A, Weinger MB, et al. Simulation for maintenance of certification in anesthesiology: the first two years. J Contin Educ Health Prof 2012;32: 236–42.
52. Weinger MB, Burden AR, Steadman RH, et al. This is not a test! Misconceptions surrounding the maintenance of certification in anesthesiology simulation course. Anesthesiology 2014;121(3):655–9.
53. Steadman RH, Burden AR, Huang YM, et al. Practice improvements based on participation in simulation for the maintenance of certification in anesthesiology program. Anesthesiology 2015;122(5):1154–69.
54. Anson JA. MOCA saves a life [letter]. ASA Newsl 2013;77(1):47.
55. Weinger MB, Banerjee A, Burden AR, et al. Simulation-based assessment of the management of critical events by board-certified anesthesiologists. Anesthesiology 2017;127(3):475–89.
56. Hanscom R. Medical simulation from an insurer's perspective. Acad Emerg Med 2008;15:984–7.
57. CRICO/RMF. Clinician resources: team training. Available at: https://www.rmf. harvard.edu/Clinician-Resources/Article/2014/OR-Team-Training-Incentive Accessed June 20, 2017.
58. The Doctors Company resources. Available at: http://www.thedoctors.com. Accessed June 3, 2017.
59. DeMaria S, Levine A, Petrou P, et al. Performance gaps and improvement plans from a 5-hospital simulation programme for anaesthesiology providers: a retrospective study. BMJ Simulation Technology Enhanced Learn. 2017:bmjstel-2016. Available at: http://stel.bmj.com/.

60. Dieckmann P, Phero JC, Issenberg SB, et al. The first Research Consensus Summit of the Society for Simulation in Healthcare: conduction and a synthesis of the results. Simul Healthc 2011;6(Suppl):S1–9.
61. American College of Surgeons, Division of Education Accredited Education Institutes. enhancing patient safety through simulation. Available at: http://www.facs.org/education/accreditationprogram/requirements.html. Accessed June 20, 2017.
62. Society for Simulation in Healthcare, Council for Accreditation of Healthcare. Simulation programs informational guide for the accreditation process from the SSH Council for Accreditation of Healthcare Simulation Programs. Available at: http://ssih.org/Accreditation. Accessed November 18, 2017.
63. Davis D, O'Brien MA, Freemantle N, et al. Impact of formal continuing medical education: do conferences, workshops, rounds, and other traditional continuing education activities change physician behavior or health care outcomes? JAMA 1999;282(9):867–74.
64. Counselman FL, Carius ML, Kowalenko T, et al. The American Board of Emergency Medicine maintenance of certification summit. J Emerg Med 2015;49: 722–8.
65. Holmboe ES, Wang Y, Meehan TP, et al. Association between maintenance of certification examination scores and quality of care for Medicare beneficiaries. Arch Intern Med 2008;168:1396–403.
66. Steadman RH. Improving on reality: can simulation facilitate practice change? Anesthesiology 2010;112(4):775–6.

Developing Multicenter Registries to Advance Quality Science

 CrossMark

Laura E. Schleelein, MD*, Kathleen A. Harris, MD,
Elizabeth M. Elliott, MD

KEYWORDS

- Clinical registry • Patient registry • Quality science • Clinical database
- Quality improvement • Multicenter

KEY POINTS

- Multicenter registries, both national and international, use observational study methods to collect data that can be used to inform members on the ideal structure, process, or outcome of a measured entity.
- The data from multicenter registries can be used as an observational tool by itself or it can serve as a platform for framing research studies, clinical trials, or quality improvement projects.
- Clinical registries can be used to achieve the 6 improvement goals in health care (care that is safe, effective, patient centered, timely, efficient, and equitable) described by the Institute of Medicine.
- Registries have the unique advantage of garnering much data quickly and are especially helpful for niche populations or low-prevalence diseases.

WHY REGISTRIES?

The gold standard for generating new medical knowledge has historically been the randomized controlled trial, but not all research questions are amenable to such methodology. Although clinical trials provide important sources of new knowledge, they may fail to yield comprehensive data sets that accurately reflect entire populations because patients may or may not meet the inclusion criteria for participation. Furthermore, results from these studies can take years before being translated into clinical use.[1,2] There are other valid approaches to gathering new knowledge, however. For example, quality improvement (QI) science has recently advanced the use of

Disclosure Statement: All authors have no disclosures.
Department of Anesthesiology and Critical Care Medicine, Children's Hospital of Philadelphia, 34th Street and Civic Center Boulevard, Main Building, 9th Floor, Suite 9329, Philadelphia, PA 19104, USA
* Corresponding author.
E-mail address: schleelein@email.chop.edu

Plan-Do-Study-Act cycles in which the provider can quickly gather a significant amount of information on a topic by considering an intervention, testing the intervention for a short time, and analyzing the result, which then forms the basis for subsequent interventions. Clinical registries have also been used as valuable tools to answer questions that might not lend themselves to formal research studies because of cost, time, and/or ethical reasons. There are several benefits to the clinical registry as an information repository tool, ultimately lending itself to acquisition of new knowledge. Multicenter registries may be required to garner sufficient patient data for rare conditions or diseases. This article reviews the design, implementation, interpretation, and outcomes associated with patient registries and ends with some well-established examples.

Definition and Design

A *patient registry* is an organized system that uses observational study methods to collect uniform data (clinical and other) to evaluate specified outcomes for a population defined by a particular disease, condition, or exposure and that serves one or more predetermined scientific, clinical, or policy purposes. The *patient registry database* describes a file (or files) derived from the registry.[3]

Many factors must be considered before a clinical registry can be formed. Key steps that should be included in the formation of a registry are as follows:

Why form a registry

- Define the purpose.
- Determine whether a registry is an appropriate means for addressing the purpose.

Who should be involved

- Identify the stakeholders.
- Assess the feasibility of forming the registry and secure funding.

What is needed

- Define the scope and target population.
- Plan for what data will be collected and how it will be collected.

How will it be maintained

- Plan for registry governance and oversight.[3,4]

There is an increasing global trend to use registry data to inform decision-making in health care.[4] Possible uses include, but are not limited to, the following[2,5–8]:

- Patient recruitment: Recruit patients for clinical trials.
- Knowledge dissemination: Distribute information on new therapies, best practices, and safety issues.
- Clinical epidemiology: Learn about population behavior patterns and their association with disease development.
- Clinical effectiveness: Develop therapeutics and assess the effects.
- Drive research: Develop research hypotheses.
- Quality and outcomes improvement: Improve and monitor the quality of health care.
- Define clinical excellence: Study best practices in care or treatment.
- Public health planning: Register the causes of disease to illustrate the need for a prevention program.

Registries are especially helpful for niche populations, chronic disease, or low-prevalence diseases whereby it is difficult to conduct large-scale studies. They can be intervention based or disease based.[3,4] An intervention-based registry addresses questions regarding appropriate use, effectiveness, cost-effectiveness, and safety. Disease-based registries facilitate studying a full disease course and treatment pathways. The type of data elements to collect depend on the goal of the registry. If the goal is to provide information on overall cost-effectiveness, for example, comprehensive data are needed on the disease, treatment, and outcomes. On the other hand, if single-outcome efficacy of an intervention is the goal, a more selective set of data elements can be collected. An analysis plan should take into account these considerations and be in place before embarking on data collection.[4]

In 2001, the Institute of Medicine issued a report, entitled Crossing the Quality Chasm, which sought to establish aims for the twenty-first century health care system. They established these improvement goals in 6 dimensions because they noted that health care today functions at far lower levels than it should in these areas. Health care should be

- *Safe*: avoiding injuries to patients from the care that is intended to help them
- *Effective*: providing services based on scientific knowledge to all who could benefit and refraining from providing services to those not likely to benefit (avoiding underuse and overuse, respectively)
- *Patient-centered*: providing care that is respectful of and responsive to individual patient preferences, needs, and values and ensuring that patient values guide all clinical decisions
- *Timely*: reducing waits and sometimes harmful delays for both those who receive and those who give care
- *Efficient*: avoiding waste, including waste of equipment, supplies, ideas, and energy
- *Equitable*: providing care that does not vary in quality because of personal characteristics, such as sex, ethnicity, geographic location, and socio-economic status[9]

Many single-institution centers are now incorporating these 6 quality dimensions when trying to deliver high-performance health care, assess quality, prioritize improvement goals, and direct resources.[10] These dimensions can also be applied and achieved when using national and international clinical registries. The nature and purpose of a registry inherently addresses most of these improvement domains and, depending on the questions posed, can involve all 6 domains. They are *safe* in that they collect data for the sole purpose of improvement in the delivery of health care. They are *effective* in that they can assimilate scientific knowledge easier for rare disease populations because of higher patient volumes in the national or international arena compared with single centers. This knowledge can then be spread to the entire population. They are *timely* and *efficient* by nature in that they do not waste time and energy in gathering data. Multicenter registries can collect information on a larger population than a single institution could in the same amount of time. They are *equitable* by nature because they can be used to break down barriers by comparing and contrasting the care, outcomes, or treatment plans for populations from different geographic locations or different socioeconomic statuses in an effort to standardize. Depending on the how the data are used, registries can be *patient centered* if the data are used, for example, for QI purposes and patients or families are included in these initiatives.

Difference between clinical trial and clinical registry It is important to highlight that registry data do not prove cause and effect; but they can reveal associations and questions that can then be answered by research studies, clinical trials, or further evaluated by QI projects.[5] The distinction between clinical registries and clinical trials is important. A registry is observational and does not specify treatments or therapies intended to change patient outcomes. In contrast, a trial involves an active intervention intended to change an outcome.[3]

Implementation

Different types of databases within the registries

There are several different classifications of data sets: fully identified, limited, and deidentified. The level of identifiable patient information is what drives the regulation process regarding collection, storing, use, and sharing of the data. Collection of data that includes patient identifiers is considered human subjects research and is regulated under the Federal Policy for the Protection of Research Subjects (Common Rule).[11] Data are exempt from the regulatory requirements of this Common Rule if the subjects cannot be identified by the information in the data set. Based on the level of deidentification, a data set can then be limited or fully deidentified. These terms are described in more detail next.

The term *identifier* means one or more data element that renders the subjects readily identifiable, also known as protected health information (PHI). The Health Insurance Portability and Accountability Act (HIPAA) includes a Standards for Privacy of Individually Identifiable Health Information (Privacy Rule) provision detailing which specific information is PHI and specifically describes what is required for deidentification of the data set.[11] There are 18 patient identifiers under the rule; if all 18 identifiers are removed, the information is considered a deidentified data set. If only certain elements remain after all others are removed, this is considered a limited data set (**Table 1**).[12,13]

Sharing information from each type of database

When sharing information with varying degrees of patient identifiers, the proper oversight must be taken to ensure the protection of the data (**Fig. 1**).

The data set can be held by a primary investigator or by an independent third-party data company that will protect and store the information (see **Fig. 1**). If the data set is deidentified, nothing further needs to take place and the information can be freely transferred between providers. If the data set has been initially collected as, or subsequently changed to, a limited data set, the recipient of the information needs a *data use agreement*. A data use agreement establishes ways in which the limited data set may be used and how it will be protected by the recipient.[12] It is a legal binding agreement between the primary provider or institution storing the data and the external entity that receives the data. The agreement delineates the confidentiality requirements, security safeguards, and the data use policy and procedures. The agreement serves both as a means of informing data users of these requirements and as a means of obtaining their agreement to abide by these requirements.[14] If the data set is fully identified, it is governed by the rules of the human subject research.

Protection of sensitive information

Depending on the registry and the data being collected, it may contain subjective and potentially sensitive information regarding liability. This circumstance has made the development of registries difficult in the past, as potential members worry about reputation, confidentiality, and legal retribution.[15] This serious concern conflicts and inhibits the valuable learning and improvements that a registry can offer. In 2005, congress passed the Patient Safety and Quality Improvement Act authorizing the creation of

Table 1
Deidentified and limited data set definitions

Data Element	Deidentified Data Set[a]	Limited Data Set
Names	Remove	Remove
Address, city, and other geographic information smaller than a state	Remove	Remove postal address information other than city, town, state, or zip code
All elements of dates (except year) including age, date of admission, date of service, date of discharge	Remove	May be included
Telephone numbers	Remove	Remove
Fax numbers	Remove	Remove
Electronic mail addresses	Remove	Remove
Social security numbers	Remove	Remove
Medical record numbers	Remove	Remove
Health plan beneficiary numbers	Remove	Remove
Account numbers	Remove	Remove
Certificate/license numbers	Remove	Remove
Vehicle identification numbers and serial numbers, including license plate numbers	Remove	Remove
Device identifiers (eg, implanted medical devices) and serial numbers	Remove	Remove
Web URLs	Remove	Remove
Internet protocol (IP) address numbers	Remove	Remove
Biometric indicators, including finger and voice prints	Remove	Remove
Full-face photographic images and any comparable images	Remove	Remove
Any other unique identifying number, characteristic, or code except as permitted earlier	Remove[b]	May be included

[a] Even if all the information listed is removed, if the provider knows that any remaining information in the data set could be used to reidentify patients, then the data set is not considered deidentified.
[b] If links must be maintained in the data set for potential later reidentification, they must be completely unrelated to any of the aforementioned elements. A subject code that reflects the order in which subjects were enrolled into a trial would be permitted.
Data from Children's Hospital of Philadelphia Institutional Review Board. Sharing Data. Available at: https://irb.research.chop.edu/sharing-data. Accessed July 14, 2017 and Guidance Regarding Methods for De-identification of Protected Health Information in Accordance with the Health Insurance Portability and Accountability Act (HIPAA) Privacy Rule. Available at: https://www.hhs.gov/hipaa/for-professionals/privacy/special-topics/de-identification/index.html. Accessed December 13, 2017.

patient safety organizations (PSOs). A PSO receives protection under this act in the form of federal confidentiality. That is to say, the data, information, discussions, and learnings that come under a PSO are protected from criminal, civil, administrative, or disciplinary proceedings.[15,16] This protection has allowed registries to form more easily and contributing members to feel more at ease and willing to be transparent.

Innovative ways to obtain complete data
One of the most important caveats in any registry is to know the denominator for the population that is being collected. This will allow for rates to be calculated in order to

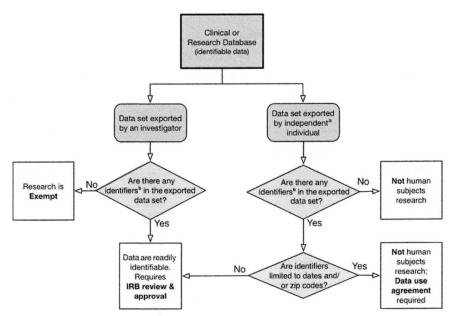

Fig. 1. Sharing data/specimens stored with identifiers. [a] *Independent* means not connected in any way to the original research, in other words, the individual is an "honest broker." [b] *Identifier* means one or more data element that renders the subjects readily identifiable. IRB, Institutional Review Board. (*From* Children's Hospital of Philadelphia Institutional Review Board. Sharing data. Available at: https://irb.research.chop.edu/sharing-data. Accessed July 14, 2017; with permission.)

quantify the issue and gives the ability to track progress. Without an accurate denominator, improvement efforts become difficult because the data is merely anecdotal and comparisons cannot be made. It is well known that capture via voluntary reporting is often deficient and not inclusive because it is labor intensive and time consuming.[17–19] There are some registries that have unique approaches to ensure the data are accurate, all inclusive, and comprehensive. The Dutch National Breast Implant Registry is now an opt-out registry, and the data are automatically entered. A prior registry was opt-in but failed to capture up to 80% of patients. This new registry not only gives necessary denominator data for breast implants in the country but it also allows for dynamic data and gives a real-time picture of hospital participation. It enables benchmarking for surgeons and plastic surgery clinics to compare themselves with the aggregated data.

Other registries are including reporting criteria in the rules of engagement and outlining the requirements for each institution to be a good citizen within the registry. The Pediatric Difficult Airway registry, for example, requires that each institution perform at a level of 90% or greater for their difficult airway capture. The registry dedicates one full-time employee specifically for auditing to make sure each site is reporting and that each report is accurate and to help with process issues.

Standardization and using the data

As registries gained popularity and the numbers of different registries started increasing, one issue with them soon became apparent. Many registries started to collect information without the consideration of how the data would be used or shared. As a result, some registries had data that were not openly available for all investigators and many were established on different operating platforms using different technology limiting interoperability. This unwillingness or inability to fully share and exchange the valuable data, experiences, and knowledge was a disappointment in the community and was ironically contrary to the original purpose of a registry.[20] As a result, the Office of Rare Diseases Research (ORDR) sponsored a 2-day workshop that was attended by several hundred experts in an effort to come to a consensus on how the registry community could standardize itself and make the data more transparent and useful. One important achievement that came out of that international meeting was the formation of a Global Rare Diseases Patient Registry Data Repository (GRDR) at the ORDR at the National Center for Advancing Translational Sciences (NCATS). The main goal of the National Institute of Health (NIH)/NCATS GRDR program is to serve as a central Web-based global data repository to integrate deidentified patient clinical data in a standardized manner to make it available to all investigators.[20,21] The first step toward this goal was to develop a set of common data elements (CDEs), which are standardized terms and data collection tools in order to allow for interoperability between databases. The NIH then expanded the CDEs to also include CDE tools that are targeted to particular disorders to obtain more granular and relevant data specific to certain diseases. The disease-specific CDEs cover domains such as neurologic disorders, substance abuse, and ophthalmic diseases.[22] Once CDEs became mainstream, the use and potential of registries exploded, with the potential to be expanded internationally.

The standardization continued even further when in 2012 the Agency for Healthcare Research and Quality formed the Registry of Patient Registries to provide a resource that was a searchable database for any patient registry in the United States.[2,23] This resource included registries not only for patient diseases but also other registries involving drugs, devices, and biological specimens.

Interpretation and Outcomes

Defining and assessing quality

How one assesses quality and improvement in health care from a clinical registry is both an interesting and difficult question. The quality of a registry is defined by the perspective of the person or group involved with the registry. This definition differs from the perspective of the health care provider, the patients, the owner of the registry, the community that the registry effects, and so forth. It is important to consider which perspective is being considered first before making conclusions about the value or success of a registry. For example, most registries are formed and run by health care professionals, which has made patients and families feel voiceless in the past. For this reason, in the mid-1990s, patients, family advocates, and organizations started creating and operating patient-powered patient registries. These registries are managed by patients and family members themselves. As a result, it gives patients and families the ability to control the agenda for using the data and/or the translation and dissemination of the research from the data.[2] The patient-powered patient registries created a venue for patients and families to feel empowered, which increased satisfaction.

The quality of a registry can also be assessed from the perspective of the structure, processes, or outcomes that it tries to measure. Registries, and health care in general, commonly use outcomes as a validation of quality. One of the main weaknesses in solely using an outcome quality indicator is it does not give insight into the strengths and weaknesses in the care that was delivered to achieve that outcome. Process evaluation can supplement outcome data because it describes the interactions between health care providers and patients. This information is often times more difficult to evaluate and describe, but it is tremendously useful because it can characterize the best practice that is associated with a desired outcome. Lastly, structure defines the number and type of resources and qualifications of clinical staff. This information is important to evaluate because more resources do not always mean better resources.[10]

A FEW EXAMPLES OF USING REGISTRY DATA
Adjunct in Quality Improvement Science

There are 4 elements that one must apply in order to conduct any QI initiative, including those that use a clinical registry. The 4 components are: appreciation of a system, understanding variation, action learning, and change management.[15,24] A system is an interdependent group working together toward a common purpose, which is key to successful QI. Understanding the variation in the system is imperative and involves QI statistics to understand normal (expected) variation versus special cause variation that is not part of the normal process and requires intervention. Action learning in QI parallels the scientific method of aim, hypothesis, study design, and experimentation. The framework for this is laid out in a key driver diagram, which consists of a smart aim or change goal, followed by key drivers or hypotheses and lastly interventions that will be tested. Change management embodies the disciplines of leadership and how to lead systems and people in change. Registry data can be used during any or all of these steps in a QI initiative. It can directly contribute to the learning during the first 3 components in any QI project. For example, the Pediatric Craniofacial Surgery Perioperative Registry has been used by the Pediatric Craniofacial Collaborative Group to evaluate the current practice with their population. After evaluation, it was concluded that blood transfusion was the norm for the patients analyzed. The group addressed the fact that surgical technique may account for some of the variability in blood product transfusion but identified the administration of antifibrinolytics as a possible intervention to improve outcomes and decrease blood loss necessitating transfusions.[25] To this end, the PCSP registry has also been used to study the safety of antifibrinolytics in pediatric cranial vault reconstruction surgery.[26] Change management is a slow process that depends on the leadership of the project, but registries can also be helpful during this phase to offer feedback regarding the intended change and if it was successful or not.

Adjunct in Randomized Controlled Trials

Registries can further advance quality science by serving as a patient base for multicenter, prospective, randomized clinical trials, such as the *Influenza Vaccination After Myocardial Infarction* (IAMI) trial.[27] There are data to suggest that the risk of myocardial infarction increases after infection with influenza. Additionally, there are small studies indicating the influenza vaccine confers some protection against future cardiac events in patients with cardiac disease; but this will be the first large-scale study to evaluate the influenza vaccine in patients with established cardiac disease. Registry data on patients presenting to hospitals in Sweden and Denmark for coronary angiography or percutaneous coronary intervention for myocardial infarction (ST-elevation myocardial infarction [STEMI]/non-STEMI) are being collected and will be used to recruit patients who present during the flu season who would otherwise not request the influenza vaccine. Patients will be randomized to receive the vaccine or placebo during their hospitalization for myocardial infarction. Primary end points for IAMI are the time to all-cause death, hospitalization for new myocardial infarction, or stent thrombosis within the first year after intervention. This study could not be possible without the identification of the patient base from the registry.

Guiding Therapy

One of the most well-known successful registries has been the cystic fibrosis (CF) registry created and managed by the Cystic Fibrosis Foundation since 1966. The initial stated goal for the Cystic Fibrosis Foundation Patient Registry (CFFPR) was to describe the CF population and track survival. Early work from the registry primarily focused on reporting descriptive data, such as lung function measurements in cohorts over time.[28] These data were incredibly valuable because it is well known that the rate of decline of the forced expiratory volume in 1 second is a key to interpreting therapeutic results, because its slowing or reversal is one of the main outcomes for therapies directed at restoring lung function.[5]

Then, in the mid 1980's, the collection capabilities of the CFFPR were expanded to start to include detailed data on complications, treatment practices, and pulmonary and nutritional outcomes.[29] It has evolved to now include more than 300 unique variables on each patient. It was recognized that the registry could be used for questions surrounding the pathogenesis of the disease, risk factors of the disease course, and outcomes. This evolution then allowed for the registry to be used not only for clinical studies but also for QI initiatives, as centers could be evaluated for practice patterns and outcomes. The success of the CFFPR has led other countries to form their own registries, which has allowed for international comparisons.[28] The possibilities are endless, as now it is possible to compare different care models or treatment approaches in different countries while taking into consideration issues like socioeconomic factors. For example, an international comparison between the Boston and Toronto centers demonstrated the ground-breaking benefits of high-fat, high-calorie diets for these patients.[30]

Describing Rare Diseases

A rare disease registry is the North American Malignant Hyperthermia Registry (NAMHR), which has been used extensively to advance knowledge about malignant hyperthermia (MH). MH is a rare disease that has a variable presentation and many nonspecific signs, symptoms, and laboratory findings. As a result, characterization of the disease is difficult and historically depends on case reports. The NAMHR was initiated in 1987 to collect data on possible MH events and use these data for advancement of quality science regarding MH. The registry data were used to verify the accuracy of the clinical grading scale that was developed to predict MH susceptibility during an event.[31] The MH clinical grading scale was then used with NAMH registry data to define the sensitivity and specificity of the caffeine-halothane contracture test, the gold standard of diagnosis.[32] The registry has also been used to define MH in subpopulations to identify underlying causes and medical conditions associated with the disease[33] and make the case for more rigorous temperature monitoring during an anesthetic to improve the chances for surviving an MH event.[34,35]

Practice Patterns and Adverse Events

The Pediatric Sedation Research Consortium (PSRC) receives data from 41 institutions, representing care provided by anesthesiologists, pediatric anesthesiologists, pediatric emergency medicine physicians, critical care physicians, nurse practitioners, physician assistants, nurses, radiologists, and dentists in non–operating room locations. The data are gathered prospectively. In a publication from 2016, the PSRC analyzed data for 57,227 patients aged 0 to 22 years to evaluate adverse events in former preterm children (<37 weeks' gestational age) versus full term. Although their data lack granularity to determine the degree of prematurity, the data did show a higher adverse event rate for any child with a history of prematurity (14.7% vs 8.5%).[36] Because the data include such a broad sampling of patients, adverse events were common enough to make associations that would have otherwise been too difficult to detect in a prospective trial with a smaller and less random sample.[37]

SUMMARY

The benefits of registries are numerous and expanding all the time as more and more barriers are broken down and the boundaries are now pushed to international limits. The Institute of Medicine has delineated 6 improvement domains for health care today. They state that health care should be safe, effective, patient centered, timely, efficient, and equitable. Registries are a helpful tool to accomplish improvement in these areas. They can be used to obtain much information on a topic in a short time and can answer several different questions depending on what is collected. The limits of what one center can collect are no longer an issue as national and international registries take hold. With proper oversight regarding storage and sharing of the data, registry data can be used anywhere from understanding disease epidemiology to advancing research initiatives or performing QI projects.

REFERENCES

1. Schoenfeld AJ, Redberg RF. The value of using registries to evaluate randomized clinical trial study populations. JAMA Intern Med 2017;177(6):889.
2. Workman TA. Engaging patients in information sharing and data collection: the role of patient-powered registries and research networks. AHRQ community forum white paper. AHRQ Publication No. 13-EHC124-EF. Rockville (MD): Agency for Healthcare Research and Quality; 2013. p. 1–14.
3. Gliklich RE, Dreyer NA. Registries for evaluating patient outcomes: a user's guide. AHRQ Publication No. 07-EHC001-1. Rockville (MD): Agency for Healthcare Research and Quality; 2007.
4. de Groot S, van der Linden N, Franken MG, et al. Balancing the optimal and the feasible: a practical guide for setting up patient registries for the collection of real-world data for health care decision making based on Dutch experiences. Value Health 2017;20(4):627–36.
5. Salvatore D, Buzzetti R, Mastella G. An overview of international literature from cystic fibrosis registries. Part 5: update 2012-2015 on lung disease. Pediatr Pulmonol 2016;51:1251–63.
6. What is a clinical registry? National Quality Registry Network (NQRN). Available at: http://www.thepcpi.org/pcpi/media/documents/nqrn-what-is-clinical-registry.pdf. Accessed July 5, 2017.
7. Freudenheim M. Tool in cystic fibrosis fight: a registry. New York Times 2009;D1.
8. Forrest CB, Bartek RJ, Rubinstein Y, et al. The case for a global rare-diseases registry. Lancet 2011;377:1057–9.
9. Institute of Medicine. Committee on quality health care in America. Crossing the quality chasm- a new health system for the 21st century. Washington, DC: National Academy Press; 2001. p. 5–6.
10. Varughese AM, Hagerman NS, Kurth CD. Quality in pediatric anesthesia. Paediatr Anaesth 2010;20:684–96.
11. Rothstein MA. Is deidentification sufficient to protect health privacy in research? Am J Bioeth 2010;10(9):3–11.
12. Sharing data. In: Children's Hospital of Philadelphia Institutional Review Board. Available at: https://irb.research.chop.edu/sharing-data. Accessed July 14, 2017.
13. De-identified data sets and limited data sets. In: University of Michigan Health System. Available at: http://www.ehcca.com/presentations/HIPAA7/4_04H2.pdf. Accessed July 25, 2017.

14. Practices guide: data use agreement. In: Department of Health and Human Services Enterprise Performance Life Cycle Framework. Available at: https://www.hhs.gov/ocio/eplc/EPLC Archive Documents/55-Data Use Agreement (DUA)/eplc_dua_practices_guide.pdf. Accessed July 14, 2017.
15. Kurth CD, Tyler D, Heitmiller E, et al. National pediatric anesthesia safety quality improvement program in the United States. Anesth Analg 2014;119(1):112–21.
16. Patient Safety Organization (PSO). In: Center for Patient Safety. Available at: http://www.centerforpatientsafety.org/pso/. Accessed July 14, 2017.
17. Leape LL. Reporting of adverse events. N Engl J Med 2002;347(20):1633–8.
18. Sanborn KV, Castro J, Kuroda M, et al. Detection of intraoperative incidents by electronic scanning of computerized anesthesia records. Comparison with voluntary reporting. Anesthesiology 1996;85(5):977–87.
19. Cooper JB. Is voluntary reporting of critical events effective for quality assurance? Anesthesiology 1996;85(5):961–4.
20. Rubinstein YR, McInnes P. NIH/NCATS/GRDR common data elements: a leading force for standardized data collection. Contemp Clin Trials 2015;42:78–80.
21. Rubinstein YR, Groft SC, Bartek R, et al. Creating a global rare disease patient registry linked to a rare diseases biorepository database: rare disease-HUB (RD-HUB). Contemp Clin Trials 2010;31:394–404.
22. Sheehan J, Hirschfeld S, Foster E, et al. Improving the value of clinical research through the use of common data elements. Clin Trials 2016;13(6):671–6.
23. Gliklich RE, Levy D, Karl J, et al. Registry of Patient Registries (RoPR): project overview. AHRQ Pulication No. 12-EHC058-EF. Rockville (MD): Agency for Healthcare Research and Quality; 2012.
24. Kurth CD. Introducing quality improvement. Paediatr Anaesth 2013;23(7):569–70.
25. Stricker PA, Goobie SM, Cladis FP, et al. Perioperative outcomes and management in pediatric complex cranial vault reconstruction: a multicenter study from the Pediatric Craniofacial Collaborative Group. Anesthesiology 2017;126(2):276–87.
26. Goobie SM, Cladis FP, Glover CD, et al. Safety of antifibrinolytics in cranial vault reconstructive surgery: a report from the Pediatric Craniofacial Collaborative Group. Paediatr Anaesth 2017;27(3):271–81.
27. Frobert O, Gotberg M, Angeras O, et al. Design and rationale for the Influenza Vaccination After Myocardial Infarction (IAMI) trial. A registry-based randomized clinical trial. Am Heart J 2017;189:94–102.
28. Schechter MS, Fink AK, Homa K, et al. The Cystic Fibrosis Foundation Patient Registry as a tool for use in quality improvement. BMJ Qual Saf 2014;23:i9–14.
29. Boyle MP, Sabadosa KA, Quinton HB, et al. Key findings of the US Cystic Fibrosis Foundation's clinical practice benchmarking project. BMJ Qual Saf 2014;23:i15–22.
30. Goss CH, MacNeill SJ, Quinton HB, et al. Children and young adults with CF in the USA have better lung function compared with the UK. Thorax 2015;70:229–36.
31. Larach MG, Localio AR, Allen GC, et al. A clinical grading scale to predict malignant hyperthermia susceptibility. Anesthesiology 1994;80(4):771–9.
32. Allen GC, Larach MG, Kunselman AR. The sensitivity and specificity of the caffeine-halothane contracture test: a report from the North American Malignant Hyperthermia Registry. The North American Malignant Hyperthermia Registry of MHAUS. Anesthesiology 1998;88(3):579–88.
33. Nelson P, Litman RS. Malignant hyperthermia in children: an analysis of the North American Malignant Hyperthermia Registry. Anesth Analg 2014;118(2):369–74.

34. Larach MG, Brandom BW, Allen GC, et al. Malignant hyperthermia deaths related to inadequate temperature monitoring, 2007-2012: a report from the North American Malignant Hyperthermia Registry of the Malignant Hyperthermia Association of the United States. Anesth Analg 2014;119(6):1359–66.

35. Litman RS, Flood CD, Kaplan RF, et al. Postoperative malignant hyperthermia: an analysis of cases from the North American Malignant Hyperthermia Registry. Anesthesiology 2008;109(5):825–9.

36. Havidich JE, Beach M, Dierdorf SF, et al. Preterm versus term children: analysis of sedation/anesthesia adverse events and longitudinal risk. Pediatrics 2016;137(3): e20150463.

37. Litman RS. The use of patient registries to detect risk factors of anesthesia and sedation complications. Pediatrics 2016;137(3):e20154579.

Handovers in Perioperative Care

Atilio Barbeito, MD, MPH[a],*, Aalok V. Agarwala, MD, MBA[b], Amanda Lorinc, MD[c]

KEYWORDS

- Handovers • Handoffs • Transitions of care • Safety • Perioperative

KEY POINTS

- Transitions of care during the perioperative period are complex and error prone.
- Preoperative handovers have not been as well studied but seem to have deficiencies similar to those found with other types of perioperative handovers.
- Although short intraoperative breaks may be helpful in reducing complications, end-of-shift intraoperative handovers seem to be associated with an increase in morbidity and mortality.
- Postoperative handovers are typically rife with errors and inefficiencies and may, therefore, present the greatest opportunity to improve safety around surgery.
- A standardized institutional process that allows flexibility among different units and settings, the completion of urgent tasks before information transfer, the presence of all members of the team for the duration of the handover, a structured conversation, and education in team skills and communication are common recommendations in the handover literature.

INTRODUCTION

Handovers (also called *handoffs* or *transitions of care*) may be defined as the process by which a patient, information relevant to that patient, equipment, and professional responsibility and accountability are transferred from one person or care team to another. Transferring patients from the intensive care unit (ICU) or holding room (HR) to the operating room (OR), providing a break or end-of-the-day relief for an anesthesia provider in the OR, and moving patients from the OR to the recovery unit or ICU following surgery are all examples of handovers. This process is repeated multiple

Disclosure Statement: None.
[a] Department of Anesthesiology, Duke University Medical Center, VA Healthcare System, DUMC Box 3094, Durham, NC 27710, USA; [b] Department of Anesthesia, Critical Care, and Pain Medicine, Massachusetts General Hospital, Harvard Medical School, 55 Fruit Street, GRJ 4-428, Boston, MA 02114, USA; [c] Department of Anesthesiology, Monroe Carell Jr. Children's Hospital at Vanderbilt, 2200 Children's Way, Suite 3115, Nashville, TN 37232, USA
* Corresponding author.
E-mail address: atilio.barbeito@duke.edu

Anesthesiology Clin 36 (2018) 87–98
https://doi.org/10.1016/j.anclin.2017.10.007
1932-2275/18/Published by Elsevier Inc.

anesthesiology.theclinics.com

times during each patient's hospital stay and, as is outlined here, constitutes a particular vulnerability in the way we provide care to surgical patients, opening the door to
adverse events, such as delays in diagnosis or treatment and medication errors.[1] In
this article, the authors discuss the importance of the handover process and review
the different handover types that may occur during the perioperative period. The authors also provide broad suggestions for implementing structured handovers in the
perioperative setting.

Why Are Handovers Important?

Despite our best efforts, errors continue to be common in health care. According
to recent estimates, medical error may be responsible for approximately 251,000
deaths yearly in the United States alone, representing the third leading cause of
death after heart disease and cancer.[2] Communication failure constitutes up to
70% of preventable errors, and half of these communication errors occur during
handovers.[3,4] Perioperative transitions of care are particularly challenging
because surgical patients are often critically ill and intensely monitored; the transfer of care frequently requires the physical transport of patients and associated
equipment; several disciplines are involved in the process; the environment is
commonly chaotic and noisy; and the process occurs while providers are simultaneously delivering care to the patients.[5] Therefore, interventions aimed at standardizing and improving the handover process have the potential to improve
patient safety around the time of surgery.

TYPES OF PERIOPERATIVE HANDOVERS

Handovers vary according to the delivering and receiving teams and/or locations.
Although the main principles for each transfer of care are the same, each setting presents certain unique characteristics and challenges. In this section, the authors review
the different types of perioperative handovers and summarize the relevant literature
(**Fig. 1**).

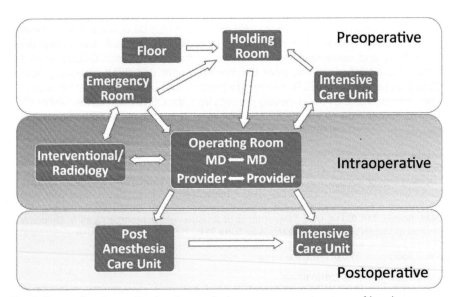

Fig. 1. Types of perioperative handovers. Each arrow represents a type of handover.

Preoperative Handovers

Holding room to operating room handovers

Most patients begin their operative course in a holding room (HR); it is here that they encounter preoperative nursing and meet their anesthesia provider and surgical team. The preoperative handover, thus, begins in the HR; yet, little information exists on these preoperative interactions. Handovers here typically involve information transfer between patients or family members, an HR nurse, an OR nurse, an anesthesia team member, and a surgical team member.

The quality and content of the information communicated in this preoperative handover varies significantly, however. One study, which followed 20 patients through their surgical course, found that although information transfer and communication failures occur across the surgical continuum, the preprocedural teamwork phase had the largest amount of failures (61.7%).[1] Although the anesthesia team had 86.6% of the necessary preoperative information and the surgical team had 82.9% of the necessary information, the nursing team only had 25% of the total information and only 27% of the total information was known by all primary team members (surgeon, anesthetist, surgical assistant, scrub tech, and circulating nurse). Verbal handover from the ward to the OR team only occurred in 43% of the patients, and in 10% of the cases there was no communication between the ward nurse and the OR team receiving the patients. They reported that information transfer failures contributed to a total of 18 incidents and adverse events in 15 out of 20 patients. In another study by Nagpal,[6] information transfer and communication failures were described in the preoperative phase. Three types of failures were described: *source failures* (information at different places, consents missing, inadequate documentation), *transmission failures* (lack of communication between anesthesia and surgical teams, lack of communication between the ward and OR staff, information not relayed), and *receiver failures* (specialists' opinions not followed, checklists not followed). These failures had effects on patients, teams, and the organization (such as case cancellations, provider stress, and wastage of resources); but these effects were not linked to particular phases of failure. Although much of this communication seems routine, 7% of anesthesia-related postanesthesia care unit (PACU) closed claims were related to preoperative preparation and communication issues, suggesting a significant unrecognized benefit in the use of structured communication in the preoperative setting.[7]

Intensive care unit to operating room handovers

Another interesting and complex transition of care, yet also vastly understudied, is ICU to OR transitions. Patients do not always arrive to the OR from an HR. They may come to the OR from any number of locations, such as the ICU, either directly or via the HR. The variability in these locations presents its own challenges and barriers, as each location may have different preparation before transfer to the OR. Team composition, policies, charting, and methods of communication may differ from unit to unit. In addition, there may be limited information available because of the emergent nature of some procedures.

In a study of neonatal ICU to OR handovers, several barriers to information exchange were discovered.[8] These barriers included a lack of a standardized report, patients not prepared for transfer, unclear transition of care between team members, unclear provider roles, provider traffic, and distractions. Not only do the providers present at the time of handover vary widely but up to 10 different providers may also be present at any given handover. In addition, the perception of handover quality varied widely, with 41% reporting fair to poor quality and only 35% reporting very good to excellent quality. Handovers in this setting need additional studies, particularly with patient-specific outcomes.

Interventions to Improve Preoperative Handovers

Because of a paucity of studies on preoperative handovers, few interventions are mentioned. In a study of pediatric HR to OR handovers, the implementation of an HR preoperative checklist revealed an underlying communication deficit, with improvement in 12 of 15 key items being discussed after implementation of the checklist.[9] Anesthesiology and preoperative nursing staff were also surveyed; 95% agreed or strongly agreed that they were satisfied with the tool, and 85% of the staff agreed or strongly agreed that the tool was efficient. The duration of handovers did not increase substantially after implementation, with most lasting 30 to 60 seconds for both preimplementation and postimplementation groups; all remained shorter than 150 seconds. Caruso showed that standardizing ICU to OR handovers increased communication without delaying surgery and improved the anesthesia provider satisfaction scores.[10] The frequency of handoffs increased from 25% to 86% (P<.0001), and the frequency of patient readiness increased from 61% to 97% (P = .001). Additional studies on preoperative handover interventions are needed.

Intraoperative Handovers

Intraoperative handovers may be temporary as for duty relief or short breaks or may be permanent as at the end of a shift. Although early work in the area suggested that intraoperative relief may have beneficial effects, more recent work has identified this critical transition of care as a potential contributor to worsened postoperative outcomes, as discussed later.

Handovers for short breaks

One of the earliest published articles on the topic of perioperative handovers was focused on the effect of intraoperative handovers on anesthesia-related adverse events. A 1982 study by Cooper and colleagues[11] reviewed more than 1000 preventable adverse events, finding 96 that involved a relief anesthetist and an intraoperative handover. Ten of 96 were incidents identified as unfavorable, with some aspect of the relief process potentially contributing to the event. However, their analysis also revealed that in 26 of the incidents, potential safety hazards were identified by the relief anesthetist, resulting in better care than may have been provided without the relief. The only other publication evaluating the effect of intraoperative breaks during anesthesia care was published nearly 35 years later, in 2016. Terekhov and colleagues[12] analyzed more than 140,000 cases at Vanderbilt University, a large academic tertiary-care hospital, finding a small, but statistically significant, 6.7% reduction in serious complications when short breaks were given during an anesthetic, despite finding no overall association between the number of intraoperative handoffs and postoperative outcomes. In thinking about why short breaks may be beneficial, it is likely that the introduction of a new provider assessing their environment for the first time leads to a fresh perspective on the clinical care plan, in addition to the ability to recognize suboptimal monitoring or other equipment malfunctions. It may also be that the ability to provide breaks is representative of other institutional factors, such as staffing and team-based care models. Although we may not know exactly why short breaks may be helpful, there has not been any evidence to date to suggest that they are harmful.

End-of-shift handovers

In contrast to findings related to short breaks, several recent studies specifically designed to examine the contribution of intraoperative handovers to patient outcomes have found cause for concern. Although each of the studies is limited by being single-center, retrospective analyses of existing large databases, 3 of 4 recent studies have found an increase in morbidity and mortality with increasing numbers of intraoperative handoffs, with one finding no association.[12] Saager and colleagues[13] used a propensity-matched study to review nearly 139,000 patients at the Cleveland Clinic and found that intraoperative handovers were associated with increased cardiac, respiratory, gastrointestinal, urinary, bleeding, and infectious complications, with each additional handover conferring an increased risk of complications of 8%. A similar, propensity-matched cohort study in more than 14,000 cardiac surgery patients at Ottawa Hospital found a 27% greater risk of major morbidity and a 43% greater risk of in-hospital mortality, with the association most pronounced in high-risk patients.[14] A smaller study at the Mayo Clinic evaluating 900 patients undergoing elective colorectal surgery found that for any given case, the odds of 30-day postoperative complications or death increased by 52% as the number of attending anesthesiologists increased.[15]

Why Might Intraoperative Handovers Lead to Poorer Outcomes?

Intraoperative handoffs are unique from other perioperative settings in that they are most often characterized by a transition of care between 2 providers with anesthesia-specific training during ongoing care of patients, though they may occur between people with varying levels and types of training (eg, attending vs certified registered nurse anesthetist vs resident). In addition, unlike preoperative and postoperative handovers, transition of equipment, monitoring, and the physical movement of patients are not generally required.

However, despite these beneficial factors, intraoperative handovers face several other challenges. They are often conducted in noisy, distraction-filled environments, often interrupted by critical patient care activities, and sometimes done in the dark. Alternatively, they may be done away from the patients, as in a hallway or over the phone. As with many other transitions of care, there is often a lack of structure to the process, resulting in significant variability between providers in what information is transferred and retained. Checklists may or may not be used, and there is rarely any formal education or training for residents and other new anesthesia providers about how to effectively handover patients.

Interventions to Improve Intraoperative Handovers

Few articles have been published addressing intraoperative handovers at all,[12,13,16–21] and even fewer have examined the effect of interventions to improve them. All of the currently available evidence focuses on the use of checklists to improve the handover process, primarily focusing on information transfer between providers. The first published proposal of a handover checklist was nearly 30 years ago by Cooper, albeit without an interventional study of whether the checklist was effective.[22] Three more recent studies, all using preinterventional-postinterventional designs, have been reported in recent years. Boat and Spaeth[20] used quality improvement techniques to implement the use of a checklist to be used for handover at the bedside, resulting in an improvement in the reliability of handovers by attending anesthesiologists. A more comprehensive study by Agarwala and colleagues[19] created and implemented a handover checklist within the electronic medical record (**Fig. 2**) for use by primary anesthetists and found significant improvements in critical information transfer and retention. The most recent study using an interventional cohort design found that training and display of a checklist for information transfer improved the quality of observed handovers by 43% as compared with a control group at a different hospital.[21]

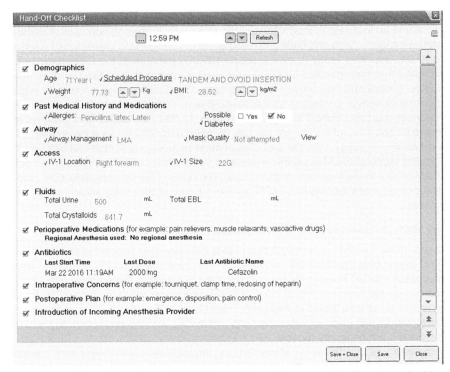

Fig. 2. An example of an electronic health record–based intraoperative handover checklist.

In summary, the available evidence about intraoperative handovers tells us 3 things:

a. Short breaks may be helpful in reducing complications and are at least unlikely to hurt.
b. Intraoperative handovers seem to be associated with an increase in morbidity and mortality.
c. The implementation of structured tools to assist with intraoperative handover can increase information transfer and retention at the time of the handover.

We do not currently have evidence regarding the impact on postoperative outcomes from these types of interventions; further investigation is necessary to elucidate not just whether but which interventions may have the greatest impact on reducing harm and improving patient safety.

Postoperative Handovers

Operating room to post anesthesia care unit handovers

Postoperative handovers are the most common and most studied handovers in anesthesiology. These typically involve anesthesia staff providing report to PACU nursing staff and may also involve surgical team members. Despite the frequency with which this handover occurs, studies have repeatedly found that the quality of the handover is variable, with many areas for improved performance. In one study of routine postoperative handovers, it was found that significant amounts of information were frequently missed, such as the American Society of Anesthesiologists' physical status, antibiotics received, and fluid management.[23] Siddiqui and colleagues[24] observed 526 handovers and found that of the 29 data items examined, only 2 items were reported in more than 90% of handovers. Handovers of ambulatory patients also commonly resulted in omission of data and resulted in poor receiver satisfaction.[25] Multitasking during handovers has been described as a common event (56%–74% of PACU handovers), but loss of information or adverse safety events were not evaluated.[26]

Studies linking poor handover quality and adverse outcomes are limited. Composites of overall handover quality have been judged to be good less than half of the time following delivery to the PACU,[27] and the variable quality of communication of pertinent case events in most postoperative handovers is associated with a significant perceived complication rate.[3,17] Data collected from the Anesthetic Incidents Monitoring Study, a voluntary, self-reporting database, revealed that 14% of 419 anesthesia-related PACU events cited failures or deficiencies in communication as a contributing factor.[7] Bittner and colleagues[28] found a correlation between increased PACU length of stay and lower-quality handovers as determined by a handover score.

Operating room to intensive care unit handovers

OR to ICU handovers have also been more commonly studied as compared with other types of perioperative handovers, perhaps because of their complexity. Surgical patients requiring postoperative ICU care are often critically ill and hemodynamically tenuous, requiring various degrees of monitoring and support in the form of mechanical ventilation and vasoactive infusions. In addition, circulatory support devices, drains and cannulas, and advanced monitoring, all commonly present in this population, make the physical transfer of patients demanding. Monitoring is typically interrupted twice, once when patients are moved from the OR table onto the ICU bed and attached to the transport monitor and then again when ICU monitoring is instituted. Furthermore, several disciplines are often involved in the transfer of care, including surgeons, anesthesiology providers, OR and ICU nurses, intensivists, and perfusionists, all with complementary but distinct needs and perspectives on the process.[29,30] All of these elements make OR to ICU handovers particularly challenging and error prone.

The literature has documented several vulnerabilities in the OR to ICU handover process. Technical errors (eg, lack of available equipment on patient arrival), failure to transfer essential information, and delays in diagnosis and treatment are all common.[31,32] For example, Joy and colleagues[32] studied pediatric cardiac surgery handovers at a single institution and showed a mean of 6.33 (95% confidence interval [CI] 5.57–7.10) information omissions and 6.24 (95% CI 5.57–6.91) technical errors per handover at baseline. McElroy and colleagues[33] performed ethnographic observations of 5 OR to ICU handovers at a tertiary academic hospital and conducted a failure modes, effects, and criticality analysis, which is a risk assessment methodology developed by the Department of Defense to assess processes in high-risk industries. Their analysis revealed 82 process failures, 22 of which were determined to be critical. Another example of the existing deficiencies with OR to ICU handovers is provided by Petrovic and colleagues.[5] They studied OR to ICU handovers in a cardiac surgical population and found, at baseline before their intervention, that none of the 30 observed handovers included all team members at the bedside simultaneously. In addition, the percentage of ICU nurses who reported that they could hear all of the report was 45% preintervention. In summary, OR to ICU handovers are complex and rife with opportunities for error.

Interventions to Improve Postoperative Handovers

There have been several studies evaluating the effects of various interventions on postoperative handovers. Salzwedel and colleagues[34] recorded and analyzed 40

PACU handovers before and 80 handovers after the implementation of a checklist, of which half were randomized to the use of the checklist and half were not. Those who used the checklist showed an increase in the number of items handed over from 32.4% to 48.7%, and this improvement was not seen in the group that received instructions about items that should be included in handovers but without the use of a checklist. There was a slight increase in the duration of handovers from 86 to 121 seconds. Structured handovers in a pediatric population have been shown to significantly decrease communication errors and increase the reliability and effectiveness of communication in the PACU.[20] Nagpal and colleagues[35] also reported a decrease in information omission and task errors and an increase in staff satisfaction after the institution of a standardized handover tool. One study showed that a multimodal intervention substantially improved PACU handovers, and the effect continued to be present 3 years after the intervention.[36] Overall, the data available support the use of a structured approach to postoperative handovers that includes a tool and education about its use. Many studies have shown interventions that improve PACU handover effectiveness, efficiency, and teamwork perception. However, additional work needs to be done to determine the effect of handover quality on patient outcomes. Two studies in the PACU population showed reductions in time to extubation and postoperative complications[37] and more timely administration of analgesia and antibiotics, with fewer hemodynamic and respiratory interventions.[38]

Regarding OR to ICU handovers, several investigators have published their interventions for improving this process. They have used diverse methods, including concepts borrowed from racing team pit crews,[39] human-centered design,[40] discussions with clinical staff,[41,42] root cause analysis,[32] and expert provider interviews,[35,43] among others. These interventions have shown a decrease in technical errors and a reduction in information omissions and improvements in efficiency (reduced handover duration), safety (fewer interruptions), provider satisfaction, and perceived teamwork. The translation of these benefits into improved clinical outcomes has been more difficult to prove. One study in a neurosurgical ICU also showed reduced ventilation duration,[41] and 2 groups demonstrated reductions in unplanned extubations and ventilator times[31] and reduced perioperative complications following cardiac surgery after the implementation of a structured OR to ICU handover process.[44]

In general, recommendations for improving OR to ICU handovers are similar to those for OR to PACU handovers: implementation of a standardized handover bundle (protocol), the use of cognitive aids, and education programs on the topic of handovers and teamwork. Unfortunately, important information regarding how these interventions were implemented is often lacking in these reports. This information is critical, as different health care systems and units typically have unique cultures, policies, team compositions, and processes of care. These differences likely influence the way handover processes should be implemented, yet little guidance exists in this respect. The Handoffs and Transitions in Critical Care (HATRICC) study, an ongoing hybrid effectiveness-implementation study of OR to ICU handovers, may be the first to provide a template for implementing this complex intervention and evaluating its effectiveness.[45]

PRACTICAL RECOMMENDATIONS FOR IMPLEMENTING A STRUCTURED HANDOVER PROCESS IN THE PERIOPERATIVE PERIOD

Each one of the perioperative handover types presented in this article will require some variation in the way patients and information are transferred among care teams.

> **Box 1**
>
> **Practical recommendations for implementing a structured handover process in the perioperative period**
>
> 1. Standardize the handover process across the institution (general format should be the same but should allow customization for each unit).
> 2. Complete urgent clinical tasks before the information transfer.
> 3. Structure the information transfer:
>   - Allow only patient-specific discussions during the verbal handovers.
>   - Use a cognitive aid (eg, checklists).
>   - Create an opportunity for providers to ask and answer questions.
>   - Require that all relevant team members be present for the duration of the handover.
> 4. Provide training in team skills and communication for staff and trainees.

Despite these differences, there are some recommendations that are common to all perioperative handovers (**Box 1**).[30,46] These recommendations include

1. Standardizing the handover process: A standardized handover process improves task performance and is generally accompanied by improved staff satisfaction. In addition, standardization places equal value on all team members and reduces the team hierarchy, resulting in improved psychological safety.
2. Completing urgent clinical tasks (such as the physical transfer of the patient and monitors) *before* the information transfer: Waiting on all team members to be ready for the information transfer portion of the handover may help reduce information omissions.
3. Structuring the information transfer: Key recommendations for this aspect of the process include the following:
   - Allow only patient-specific discussions during verbal handovers (sterile cockpit).
   - Use a cognitive aid (eg, checklists; see **Fig. 2** for examples).
   - Create an opportunity for providers to ask and answer questions.
   - Require that all relevant team members be present for the duration of the handover.
4. Providing training in team skills and communication: The Accreditation Council for Graduate Medical Education requires that residency programs maintain formal educational programs in handovers and care transitions.[47]

SUMMARY

Transitions of care during the perioperative period are complex and error prone. Pre-operative handovers (preoperative HR to the OR, and ICU to OR) have not been as well studied but seem to have deficiencies similar to those found with other types of perioperative handovers and, thus, may benefit from standardized protocols. Although the provision of short intraoperative breaks may be helpful in reducing complications, end-of-shift intraoperative handovers seem to be associated with an increase in morbidity and mortality. Postoperative handovers have been the most studied and may present the greatest opportunity to improve safety around surgery. Interventions aimed at improving these processes have shown such benefits as increased provider satisfaction and teamwork, improved efficiency, and improved communication and have been shown to reduce errors and improve clinical outcomes. A standardized institutional process that allows flexibility among different units and settings, the completion of urgent tasks before information transfer, the presence of all members of the team for the duration of the handover, a structured conversation that uses a cognitive aid, and education in team skills and communication are common recommendations in the handover literature.

REFERENCES

1. Nagpal K, Vats A, Ahmed K, et al. An evaluation of information transfer through the continuum of surgical care: a feasibility study. Ann Surg 2010;252(2):402–7.
2. Makary MA, Daniel M. Medical error-the third leading cause of death in the US. BMJ 2016;353:i2139.
3. Choromanski D, Frederick J, McKelvey GM, et al. Intraoperative patient information handover between anesthesia providers. J Biomed Res 2014;28(5):383–7.
4. Lane-Fall MB, Brooks AK, Wilkins SA, et al. Addressing the mandate for hand-off education: a focused review and recommendations for anesthesia resident curriculum development and evaluation. Anesthesiology 2014;120(1):218–29.
5. Petrovic MA, Aboumatar H, Baumgartner WA, et al. Pilot implementation of a perioperative protocol to guide operating room-to-intensive care unit patient handoffs. J Cardiothorac Vasc Anesth 2012;26(1):11–6.
6. Nagpal K, Arora S, Vats A, et al. Failures in communication and information transfer across the surgical care pathway: interview study. BMJ Qual Saf 2012;21(10):843–9.
7. Kluger MT, Bullock MF. Recovery room incidents: a review of 419 reports from the Anaesthetic Incident Monitoring Study (AIMS). Anaesthesia 2002;57(11):1060–6.
8. Lorinc A, Roberts D, Slagle J, et al. Barriers to effective preoperative handover communication in the neonatal intensive care unit. Proc Hum Factors Ergon Soc Annu Meet 2014;58(1):1285–98.
9. Lorinc A, Crotts C, Sullivan M, et al. Pediatric preoperative handovers: does a checklist improve information exchange? ASA 2016.
10. Caruso TJ, Marquez JLS, Gipp MS, et al. Standardized ICU to OR handoff increases communication without delaying surgery. Int J Health Care Qual Assur 2017;30(4):304–11.
11. Cooper JB, Long CD, Newbower RS, et al. Critical incidents associated with intraoperative exchanges of anesthesia personnel. Anesthesiology 1982;56(6):456–61.
12. Terekhov MA, Ehrenfeld JM, Dutton RP, et al. Intraoperative care transitions are not associated with postoperative adverse outcomes. Anesthesiology 2016;125(4):690–9.
13. Saager L, Hesler BD, You J, et al. Intraoperative transitions of anesthesia care and postoperative adverse outcomes. Anesthesiology 2014;121(4):695–706.
14. Hudson CC, McDonald B, Hudson JK, et al. Impact of anesthetic handover on mortality and morbidity in cardiac surgery: a cohort study. J Cardiothorac Vasc Anesth 2015;29(1):11–6.
15. Hyder JA, Bohman JK, Kor DJ, et al. Anesthesia care transitions and risk of postoperative complications. Anesth Analg 2016;122(1):134–44.
16. Horn J, Bell MD, Moss E. Handover of responsibility for the anaesthetised patient - opinion and practice. Anaesthesia 2004;59(7):658–63.
17. Jayaswal S, Berry L, Leopold R, et al. Evaluating safety of handoffs between anesthesia care providers. Ochsner J 2011;11(2):99–101.
18. Tan JA, Helsten D. Intraoperative handoffs. Int Anesthesiol Clin 2013;51(1):31–42.

19. Agarwala AV, Firth PG, Albrecht MA, et al. An electronic checklist improves transfer and retention of critical information at intraoperative handoff of care. Anesth Analg 2015;120(1):96–104.

20. Boat AC, Spaeth JP. Handoff checklists improve the reliability of patient handoffs in the operating room and postanesthesia care unit. Paediatr Anaesth 2013;23(7): 647–54.

21. Jullia M, Tronet A, Fraumar F, et al. Training in intraoperative handover and display of a checklist improve communication during transfer of care: an interventional cohort study of anaesthesia residents and nurse anaesthetists. Eur J Anaesthesiol 2017;34(7):471–6.

22. Cooper JB. Do short breaks increase or decrease anesthetic risk? J Clin Anesth 1989;1(3):228–31.

23. Milby A, Bohmer A, Gerbershagen MU, et al. Quality of post-operative patient handover in the post-anaesthesia care unit: a prospective analysis. Acta Anaesthesiol Scand 2014;58(2):192–7.

24. Siddiqui N, Arzola C, Iqbal M, et al. Deficits in information transfer between anaesthesiologist and postanaesthesia care unit staff: an analysis of patient handover. Eur J Anaesthesiol 2012;29(9):438–45.

25. Pukenas EW, Deal ER, Allen E, et al. The ambulatory handoff: fast-paced, high-stakes patient care transitions. ASA Abstracts 2014;1(2).

26. van Rensen EL, Groen ES, Numan SC, et al. Multitasking during patient handover in the recovery room. Anesth Analg 2012;115(5):1183–7.

27. Anwari JS. Quality of handover to the postanaesthesia care unit nurse. Anaesthesia 2002;57(5):488–93.

28. Bittner EA, George E, Eikermann M, et al. Evaluation of the association between quality of handover and length of stay in the post anaesthesia care unit: a pilot study. Anaesthesia 2012;67(5):548–9.

29. Bonifacio AS, Segall N, Barbeito A, et al. Handovers from the OR to the ICU. Int Anesthesiol Clin 2013;51(1):43–61.

30. Segall N, Bonifacio AS, Schroeder RA, et al. Can we make postoperative patient handovers safer? A systematic review of the literature. Anesth Analg 2012;115(1): 102–15.

31. Kaufmnan J, Twite M, Barrett C, et al. A handoff protocol from the cardiovascular operating room to cardiac ICU is associated with improvements in care beyond the immediate postoperative period. Jt Comm J Qual Patient Saf 2013;39(7):306–11.

32. Joy BF, Elliott E, Hardy C, et al. Standardized multidisciplinary protocol improves handover of cardiac surgery patients to the intensive care unit. Pediatr Crit Care Med 2011;12(3):304–8.

33. McElroy LM, Collins KM, Koller FL, et al. Operating room to intensive care unit handoffs and the risks of patient harm. Surgery 2015;158(3):588–94.

34. Salzwedel C, Bartz HJ, Kuhnelt I, et al. The effect of a checklist on the quality of post-anaesthesia patient handover: a randomized controlled trial. Int J Qual Health Care 2013;25(2):176–81.

35. Nagpal K, Abboudi M, Manchanda C, et al. Improving postoperative handover: a prospective observational study. Am J Surg 2013;206(4):494–501.

36. Weinger MB, Slagle JM, Kuntz AH, et al. A multimodal intervention improves postanesthesia care unit handovers. Anesth Analg 2015;121(4):957–71.

37. Agarwal HS, Saville BR, Slayton JM, et al. Standardized postoperative handover process improves outcomes in the intensive care unit: a model for operational sustainability and improved team performance*. Crit Care Med 2012;40(7): 2109–15.

38. Breuer RK, Taicher B, Turner DA, et al. Standardizing postoperative PICU handovers improves handover metrics and patient outcomes. Pediatr Crit Care Med 2015;16(3):256–63.
39. Catchpole KR, de Leval MR, McEwan A, et al. Patient handover from surgery to intensive care: using Formula 1 pit-stop and aviation models to improve safety and quality. Paediatr Anaesth 2007;17(5):470–8.
40. Segall N, Bonifacio AS, Barbeito A, et al. Operating room-to-ICU patient handovers: a multidisciplinary human-centered design approach. Jt Comm J Qual Patient Saf 2016;42(9):400–14.
41. Craig R, Moxey L, Young D, et al. Strengthening handover communication in pediatric cardiac intensive care. Paediatr Anaesth 2012;22(4):393–9.
42. Zavalkoff SR, Razack SI, Lavoie J, et al. Handover after pediatric heart surgery: a simple tool improves information exchange. Pediatr Crit Care Med 2011;12(3): 309–13.
43. Yang JG, Zhang J. Improving the postoperative handover process in the intensive care unit of a tertiary teaching hospital. J Clin Nurs 2016;25(7–8):1062–72.
44. Hall M, Robertson J, Merkel M, et al. A structured transfer of care process reduces perioperative complications in cardiac surgery patients. Anesth Analg 2017;125(2):477–82.
45. Lane-Fall MB, Beidas RS, Pascual JL, et al. Handoffs and transitions in critical care (HATRICC): protocol for a mixed methods study of operating room to intensive care unit handoffs. BMC Surg 2014;14:96.
46. Nagpal K, Abboudi M, Fischler L, et al. Evaluation of postoperative handover using a tool to assess information transfer and teamwork. Ann Surg 2011;253(4): 831–7.
47. Accreditation Council for Graduate Medical Education. Program director guide to the common program requirements. 2017. Available at: http://www.acgme.org/acgmeweb/tabid/429/ProgramandInstitutionalAccreditation/CommonProgramRequirements.aspx. Accessed August 12, 2017.

Rethinking Clinical Workflow

Joseph J. Schlesinger, MD[a,*], Kendall Burdick, BS[b], Sarah Baum, PhD[c],
Melissa Bellomy, MD[d], Dorothee Mueller, MD[a], Alistair MacDonald, MD[e],
Alex Chern, PhD[f], Kristin Chrouser, MD[g], Christie Burger, PharmD[h]

KEYWORDS

- Workflow • Team dynamics • Urgency • Attention • Distractions

KEY POINTS

- Clinical workflow is modulated via models interpolating human factors to neural processing.
- Music perception and cognition research translates into clinical workflow principles of urgency and attention.
- Work system, process, and outcomes can only be improved through understanding the organization, physical environment, person, tasks, technology, and tools.

WORKFLOW, TEAM DYNAMICS, AND CLINICAL ENVIRONMENTS

As the demands and expectations of the modern world change, industries and workflow must also adapt. Because of the complex nature of so many industries (health care is just one example) the process for rethinking workflow must be as complex as the nature of the workflow itself. For high consequence industries, such as health care, aviation, and nuclear power, rethinking and optimizing workflow requires the integration of a detailed and consistently reanalyzed improvement plan. These plans are formulated from several historically successful improvement techniques, such as the Plan-Do-Check-Act (PDCA) cycle, Six Sigma, and Crew Resource Management.

There are absolutely no conflicts of interest from any author for this submission whatsoever.
[a] Department of Anesthesiology, Division of Critical Care Medicine, Vanderbilt University Medical Center, 1211 21st Avenue South, Medical Arts Building, Suite 422, Nashville, TN 37212, USA; [b] Neuroscience/Pre-Med Undergraduate, Vanderbilt University, 1211 21st Avenue South, Medical Arts Building, Suite 422, Nashville, TN 37212, USA; [c] Institute for Learning and Brain Sciences, University of Washington, 1715 NE Columbia Road, Seattle, WA 98195, USA; [d] Department of Anesthesiology, Vanderbilt University Medical Center, 1211 21st Avenue South, Medical Arts Building, Suite 422, Nashville, TN 37212, USA; [e] St. Patrick's Hospital, 500 West Broadway, Missoula, MT 59802, USA; [f] Vanderbilt University Medical Center, 1211 21st Avenue South, Medical Arts Building, Suite 422, Nashville, TN 37212, USA; [g] Department of Urology, University of Minnesota, 720 University Ave SE, Minneapolis, MN 55414, USA; [h] VA Tennessee Valley Healthcare System, 1310 24th Avenue S, Nashville, TN 37212, USA
* Corresponding author.
E-mail address: joseph.j.schlesinger@vanderbilt.edu

Anesthesiology Clin 36 (2018) 99–116
https://doi.org/10.1016/j.anclin.2017.10.008
1932-2275/18/© 2017 Elsevier Inc. All rights reserved.

anesthesiology.theclinics.com

Although each industry has formed a technique that functions the best for them, each optimization process contains aspects that mirror the founding frameworks of Taylor and Drucker. For example, the Maestro Concept is used in journalism work-rooms to encourage a project-based, team-centered workflow.[1] The goal of this work concept is to "think like the reader." The maestro role is held by the editor, who stresses teamwork and big picture thinking. In health care, this is synonymous to treatment plans that incorporate "think like the patient." A similar technique is Kaizen, meaning "change for the better."[2] Kaizen has been adopted by management systems in massive organizations, such as Toyota and the government of the Indian state of Gujarat. The Kaizen action plan and philosophy used a broad action plan (PDCA cycle) also commonly referred to as the Shewhart Cycle. Walter Shewhart began the thinking for this type of quality management, and so the established She-whart Cycle was named in his honor by W. Edwards Deming in 1993.[3] The Shewhart cycle has become so widely used that many industries use it implicitly. Health care, for example, functions as a team of providers that create a plan and actively rework it as additional data become available. This cycle provides grounds for broad and small application, while offering opportunity for continuous improvement.

Although these previous techniques and philosophies effectively encourage improvement, Six Sigma is generally regarded as the most well-known and over-arching process improvement technique; more than 100 of the largest companies in the United States have claimed success with this technique. Six Sigma is an imple-mentation method focused on minimizing error and maximizing benefits.[4] It was created to replace older top-down management styles and implement number- and error-focused reform. Six Sigma is used in such industries as health care, government, and financial services. The numbers-driven program uses proven successful ap-proaches to focus on variation reduction and process improvement to result in an operational process being virtually error free. Six Sigma was made famous by its suc-cess at General Electric, led by Jack Welch. Six Sigma created the Define, Measure, Analyze, Improve, and Control framework, a more advanced version of PDCA, to accomplish its goals. The Six Sigma approach requires first defining the consumer, measuring current performance, and then analyzing data to implement an improved process.

Six Sigma has also delivered multiple successes in the health care industry. For example, in a 2010 study, Six Sigma's Define, Measure, Analyze, Improve, and Control framework was applied to an operating room (OR) at a high-volume tertiary care med-ical center to assess process and cost efficiency.[5] The entire surgical process, from the decision to operate to discharge, was analyzed with the goals of increasing OR efficiency and financial performance across the entire operating suite. The implemen-tation of a Six Sigma program resulted in performance gains that were substantial, sustainable, financially positive, and transferrable to other specialties within the med-ical center.

Many health care locations have also adopted Six Sigma to improve efficiency and decrease error in several their safety procedures. The Six Sigma success at Massa-chusetts General Hospital (Boston, MA), Virginia Mason Medical Center (Seattle, WA), Mayo Clinic (Rochester, MN), and Clearview Cancer Institute (Huntsville, AL) was referenced at the 2009 American Society for Quality conference.[6] The Mayo Clinic's success was so significant that they created a curriculum for other health care providers to use and effectively rework their own safety measures.[7] Using Six Sigma techniques, the Mayo Clinic Quality Academy goes further than teaching pro-tocols for disease management by also incorporating topics related to quality improvement and measurement, patient safety, evidence-based medicine, and more.

HEALTH CARE–SPECIFIC WORKFLOW MODELS

Since the Institute of Medicine published the report "To err is human" in 2000 there has been a major push to re-examine the health care system, clinical work flow, and human factors to improve patient safety and prevent adverse outcomes.[8] Several of these models designed for other high-consequence industries have been adapted for health care with varying success. However, clinical workflow and the health care environment have added complexities often involving multiple personnel, roles, and processes, evolving technology, and external forces, which has led to the development of models specific to health care.[9]

HUMAN FACTORS AND THE DONABEDIAN STRUCTURE-PROCESS-OUTCOME FRAMEWORK

A subset of systems engineering known as human factors highlights the interactive nature of medicine, looking at interplay between people and their environment, safety and health, quality of working life, and the goods or services produced.[10] The Structure-Process-Outcome framework designed by Donabedian[11] describes these interactions between people and their environments to identify potential areas of improvement. Donabedian's model describes how the system (or structure) affects the safety of care provided (the process) and this process (ie, the means of caring for and managing the patient) affects patient safety (the outcome). This is a highly interactive system and changes to any one component affect the work and clinical processes of patients, employees, and organizational outcomes. Although helpful to understand the complexities of health care, one disadvantage of the Structure-Process-Outcome model is its focus on providers and their relationship with processes and outcomes rather than the structure and work systems, such as the organization or environment.

THE SYSTEMS ENGINEERING INITIATIVE FOR PATIENT SAFETY MODEL

To more fully incorporate the many systems and personnel involved in clinical workflow, Carayon and colleagues[10] at the University of Wisconsin have engineered a model titled the Systems Engineering Initiative for Patient Safety (SEIPS) (**Fig. 1**). SEIPS is a novel model of work system and patient safety, which integrates human factors and other health care quality models, such as those previously described in this article. In contrast to Donabedian's framework, the SEIPS model emphasizes structure by including systems, such as the physical climate, organizational culture and climate, error reporting and analysis, and work design, and highlighting the linkage of structures, processes, and outcomes. Additionally, the SEIPS model explains how design of the system can also affect employee and organizational outcomes, which in turn can compromise patient safety.

This model is used to guide the examination and redesign of systems and processes related to patient safety and potential or actual medical errors by specifying system components and interactions (**Table 1**), which can contribute to these undesired outcomes. By incorporating each of the elements at play, the SEIPS model demonstrates that although individual health care practitioner knowledge is important, it must also be supported by well-engineered systems and processes to ensure high-quality care and patient safety.[10] This way of thinking allows for the entire work system to be designed for optimal performance, shifting away from the previously popular practice of blaming individuals for errors and promoting a culture of safety. In addition, the SEIPS model demonstrates feedback loops from processes and outcomes back to the system/structure (see **Fig. 1**), representing pathways for system redesign.

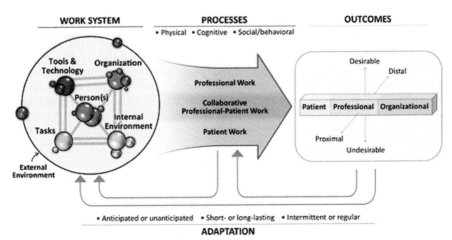

Fig. 1. SEIPS 2.0 model. (*Adapted from* Carayon P, Schoofs Hundt A, Karsh BT, et al. Work system design for patient safety: the SEIPS model. Qual Saf Health Care 2006;15(Suppl 1):i51; with permission.)

Ultimately, the goal of the SEIPS model is to provide a framework for thinking about all aspects of a work system, their interactions, and possible outcomes. These components interact with each other to influence clinical workflow and patient safety.

Given the complex nature of workflow in high consequence industries, specifically health care, a new field of human factors and clinical engineering has been developed to optimize patient safety and improve clinical workflow in the clinics, hospital wards,

Table 1		
Components of the SEIPS model		
System/structure	Technology and tools	Electronic health records, provider order entry, bar coding medication administration, medical devices, usability of tools
	Organization	Teamwork, coordination, collaboration, communication, organizational culture, work schedules, management style
	Person	Education, skills, knowledge, motivation, needs, physical ability, psychological characteristics
	Tasks	Variety of tasks, job content, challenge and use of skills, autonomy, workload, time pressure, cognitive load
	Environment	Layout, noise, lighting, temperature/humidity/air quality, work station design
Processes	Care processes	Patient care
	Other processes	Information flow, purchasing, maintenance, cleaning, process improvement activities
Outcomes	Patient outcomes	Quality of care Patient safety
	Employee outcomes	Safety, health, satisfaction, stress, burnout
	Organizational outcomes	Turnover rates, injuries and illnesses, organizational health (ie, profitability)

Adapted from Carayon P, Schoofs Hundt A, Karsh BT, et al. Work system design for patient safety: the SEIPS model. Qual Saf Health Care 2006;15(Suppl 1):i52; with permission.

intensive care units (ICUs), and ORs. This is a new field that is rapidly growing, just as its subject, medicine, continues to evolve.

URGENCY AND ATTENTION: IMPACTING CLINICAL WORKFLOW
Conveying Urgency in a Clinical Setting

The inability to effectively communicate urgency of a situation in a clinical setting often occurs when the perceived urgency conveyed by an alarm is not congruent with the actual urgency of the situation.[12] Only a small proportion of alarms signal life-threatening conditions that require a clinical response. Up to 80% to 99% of clinical alarms are false alarms; a false alarm is an alarm with no clinical or therapeutic conse-quence.[13,14] Large numbers of false alarms has led to adverse downstream conse-quences, such as disruption in patient care missed critical events, patient dissatisfaction, and unnecessary treatments.[15,16] The US Food and Drug Administra-tion Manufacturer and User Facility Device Experience database reported more than 500 alarm-related patient deaths between January 2005 and June 2010.[17] Alarms, pages, telephone calls, and other mechanisms of conveying urgency also disrupt clinical workflow; they are distracting and can have negative implications toward pa-tient outcomes.[18,19] Moreover, urgent situations are associated with increased risk because humans tend to make less accurate, less preferred, and less informed deci-sions when the time to make that decision is compressed.[20]

Culture–Societal Customs and Hierarchy in Medicine

Culture and hierarchical norms also affect the ability to communicate urgency in the context of workflow. In *Outliers*, Malcolm Gladwell suggests that Korean Air had more plane crashes than most airlines for a period in the late 1990s because of the strict hierarchical nature of Korean culture (one was expected to be deferential to elders and superiors in a way unfamiliar to people in the United States). Because mod-ern airplanes (ie, Boeing and Airbus) are intended to be flown by two equals, this pre-sents a problem if the first officer is unable to speak up to the captain.[21] Such hierarchical problems still exist in medicine. For instance, consider a situation where there is a code, and a junior resident, who knows the patient, is running the code. Later, a senior resident, who is less familiar with the patient, shows up later. Who runs the code, the junior resident who was initially present and knows the patient, or the senior resident, who knows the patient less well, but has higher rank and more medical knowledge? In the culture of medicine, where a substantial power distance can still exist between two people, it is difficult for someone lower on the pecking order (ie, a junior trainee) to speak up to someone in a higher position (ie, an attending physician), even in urgent situations.[21] Although cultural norms and hierarchy influence workflow, the initial person providing intervention (first responder), despite a relative lack of training, may have a more keen and synthetic understanding of the emergency situation.

Taking Lessons from Music Perception and Cognition

Urgency can also be approached from the angle of music perception and cognition. Individual sound parameters, such as speed, rhythm, pitch range, and melodic struc-ture, can affect the perceived urgency of an alarm.[22] Music, which is defined as an art form and cultural activity whose medium is sound organized in time, uses these ele-ments to express ideas and emotions.[23,24] Writers of music, such as composers and songwriters, are analogous to sonic chefs who combine ingredients, such as pitch, interval, harmony, and rhythm, to concoct an evocative piece of music that conveys emotion and affect, such as peace, excitement, anger, or distress. For example, the theme from the movie Jaws uses speed and loudness to communicate urgency and importance. As the shark approaches, the music becomes faster and louder, a musical Doppler effect, as it were.[25] Johann Mattheson, an eighteenth century German composer and music theorist, compiled ideas on how to create specific affects. To evoke "pride, haughtiness, and the like," Mattheson suggested one "must never permit a musical line that is, fleeting and falling, but always ascending," but to evoke joy, one should "express this affect by large and expanded [pitch] intervals."[26]

An ideal alarm should be associated with an event of clinical significance, and be easily learned and retained.[27,28] Similarly, a short, recurrent musical idea, a motif, is frequently used to create associations in musical works. Musical motifs are pervasive in daily life: jingles (persuasive multimedia), the Windows desktop music theme (computer auditory displays), and ringtones (cell phones) are all musical motifs.

The first four notes of "Dies Irae" (Day of Wrath), a thirteenth century Gregorian chant, have been quoted in musical works throughout history as a motif with connotations of fate and death (**Fig. 2**).[29] Marianne Ploger, Associate Professor of Music Perception and Cognition at the Blair School of Music at Vanderbilt University, suggests that there is an inherent quality of the motif itself that lends itself to these associations, because "each of the eleven basic intervals [in Western music] have an affective character."[30,31]

John Williams used the Wagnerian concept of leitmotif in the movie Star Wars to create associations with a specific person, place, or idea (eg, Princess Leia, Darth Vader, or the Force), consequently providing a deeper, affective understanding of the characters and themes throughout the movie.[32]

A New Interdisciplinary Approach

Urgency is a crucial element of clinical workflow given its ubiquitous presence in the clinical space, most notably in the form of alarms. Currently, urgency often is not conveyed well, because perceived urgency is not always congruent with actual urgency. The International Electrotechnical Commission 60,601-1-8 provides a standard for making distinct melodic alarms, with each representing a specific physiologic system.[33] Unfortunately, there are many reported problems with International Electrotechnical Commission alarms; they have been shown to be difficult to learn and retain and frequently confused with one another.[27,34–36] Thus, we should rethink the approach to conveying urgency in the clinical space by looking toward other fields for inspiration. High-consequence industries highlight the benefits of universal guidelines and simulation training for urgent situations. Although many studies on alarm improvement have been published, music perception and cognition allows one to approach this problem from a novel perspective. For example, Gillard and Schutz[37] explored how certain features in the musical structure of auditory alarms (ie, distinct pitch contours, repetitive notes, and easily identifiable intervals) contribute to alarm discrimination. These fields provide unique opportunities to inspire future, interdisciplinary research that may be applied to improve the design of auditory alarms, which

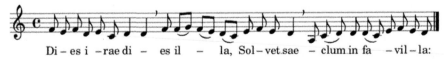

Di – es i –rae di – es il – la, Sol–vet sae – clum in fa – vil – la:

Fig. 2. Dies Irae motif. (*Data from* Dies Irae musical notation. Available at: https://en.wikipedia.org/wiki/Dies_irae#/media/File:Dies_irae.gif. Accessed June 17, 2017.)

in turn optimizes how urgency is conveyed in the clinical space and empowers one to rethink clinical workflow.

Attention and Space

The everyday environment is littered with an abundance of information. Simply navigating down a city sidewalk involves processing tactile and proprioceptive cues from our feet and body and auditory and visual cues from cars and fellow pedestrians. To successfully perceive any piece of information, there must be a process for determining what is "signal" versus "noise," and furthermore this process must be able to dynamically update based on shifting task demands.[38] The mechanisms by which one can deploy attention to preferentially process particular stimuli over others are a matter of debate within the attention literature. One line of thinking posits that attention functions like a spotlight, effectively shining light on stimuli of interest,[39] and attention then is allocated as a function of where stimuli occur within the physical space around us. This kind of attention has been well studied in the visual domain.[40] In general, the neural response to an object within the locus of spatial attention is greater than in unattended locations.[41]

Although comparatively less work has been done to examine auditory spatial attention, there is evidence to suggest that the neural mechanisms that underlie the attention to a particular part of space are similar for visual and auditory stimuli.[42,43] For example, auditory spatial attention shows a similar drop in performance when target sounds are further from the attended location.[44] Generally, attention is thought to be a supramodal process, although modality-specific effects in the alerting and orienting components of attention have been found.[45]

Auditory Scene Analysis

When viewing a perceptual scene, our perceptual system is easily able to parse all the visual elements into individual objects. A car passing on the street, for example, is identified by all the car parts moving together at the same time. Similarly, the human brain is able to bind together different auditory signals into meaningful groupings while also segregating these signals from each other and from whatever is considered background noise, a process called auditory scene analysis.[46] These signal groupings form auditory objects, such as the sound of the first violin part during the symphony, or the person standing next to you. By understanding these principles that underlie human perception, one can rethink clinical workflow by intentional training to improve neural processes, perceived urgency, attention distribution, and clinical care.

INTRAOPERATIVE DISTRACTIONS: IMPACT ON WORKFLOW AND PRODUCTIVITY

Work productivity (including quality and efficiency) is impacted by interruptions, disruptions, and distractions that are external (environment and interpersonal) and internal. In the surgical literature, the definitions and implications of distractions, diverted attention, disruptions, breaks in task, and interruptions vary, making comparing and summarizing studies challenging. For the purpose of this discussion, we focus mainly on distractions (shift in provider attention) and interruptions (pause or cessation of task) in OR workflow that introduce the potential for adverse effects on surgical quality and/or efficiency. Distractions and interruptions can negatively affect provider performance during surgery through multiple mechanisms: by impacting the overall surgical process (inefficiency), the task at hand (errors), or by generating negative emotions within providers that can lead to disruptive behavior that impacts their teams.

External Distractions

There are many external sources of disruption, distraction, and interruptions during surgery that can affect the sterile team and anesthesia providers. Both surveys and observational studies have documented the following culprits: movement (door opening or monitor obstruction/adjustment), equipment/instrument problems, team coordination, communication (relevant and nonrelevant), incoming pages/telephone calls, procedural problems, teaching, team member (or assistant) error, and ambient noise (including music).[47] The noise in many ORs exceeds recommended levels for clear verbal communication.[48] The incidence of distractions varies based on case type. Equipment and monitor issues are responsible for most interruptions during endoscopic and minimally invasive surgery, whereas case-irrelevant conversation more commonly affected open cases.[49] Failure of coordination, such as a patient being fed before surgery or the wrong patient being sent from the ward to the OR, can disrupt the flow of the surgical schedule and frustrate the entire surgical team. A recent review of surgical distractions found that overall the most frequently occurring distractions included movement (of door or monitor) and case-irrelevant conversations, whereas the most consequential distractions were equipment issues, procedural problems, and irrelevant communications.[47]

Performance Impact

Simulation studies have assessed the effects of different external distractions on intraoperative performance. A study of a laparoscopic cholecystectomy on a virtual reality simulator under artificially distracting conditions (music + irrelevant conversation) led to higher error rates and longer operative times in novices.[50] Surgeons in a simulated setting of background noise + music + a complex laparoscopic task had poor comprehension of verbal communication. Under experimentally distracting conditions (assistant's mishandling laparoscope and extraneous staff conversation), residents' technical performance decreased and their irritability increased relative to control subjects.[50] Medical students were unaware that distraction affected their performance on an endourology simulator.[51] A recent review of the effect of surgical distractions concluded that despite some inconsistency in the literature, in general novices reduce speed when distracted, whereas experienced residents and attending surgeons maintain speed but at the cost of increased errors.[47] Auditory and mental distractions seem to impair surgical performance more than visual distractions in experimental studies.[47] Observational studies in the OR have corroborated findings from the simulation laboratory. Not only do observational studies note that distractions and interruptions lead to inefficiencies, but they also negatively influence surgical performance. In observations of urologic surgeries (n = 24 cases), distractions correlated with poor intraoperative checklist compliance.[52] In cardiac surgery (n = 31 cases) error rates increased with number of disruptions.[53] In cardiac surgery (450 cases) provider-identified precursor events (including distractions) were correlated with near miss events and patient mortality.[54] In contrast, some low level distracting communication/interaction might be beneficial for anesthesia providers during maintenance to combat boredom.[55]

Internal Distractions

Although most distractions during surgery are external (from the environment or team members), distractions are also internal. Surgeons interviewed about stressful intraoperative situations recalled being distracted by worrying about the medicolegal implications of their actions, and how they would justify their actions to others postoperatively.[56] Surgeons also have high rates of musculoskeletal disorders (because of intraoperative ergonomic challenges) introducing the potential for distraction by their own physical pain, particularly during long or difficult cases.[57] The normal provider physiologic stress response to unexpected intraoperative events (eg, elevated heart rate) is uncomfortable and distracting to some individuals.[58] Many of the external distractions discussed previously can also lead to negative emotions, such as frustration, anger, irritability, anxiety, or stress in surgical providers. Such emotions are distracting, reducing the efficiency of information processing.[59] They can also spark conflict among OR team members with undesirable effects on task performance and interpersonal relationships.[60] Negative emotions can also lead to disruptive behavior, which is unfortunately common in the OR. In a survey of registered nurses, 97% (n = 244) reported witnessing disruptive behavior by surgeons in the OR, and 19% were aware of a specific adverse event associated with such behaviors.[61] In another survey of OR team members, 68% of nurses and attending surgeons and 86% of trainees admitted they were more likely to make errors in tense or hostile environments (n = 352).[62] Until recently only survey and qualitative evidence linked negative interpersonal interactions with performance. However, a recent randomized trial of neonatal resuscitation simulation found diagnostic, procedural, and information sharing scores lower in teams who heard rude comments by a colleague, even when not directed at them personally.[63] The authors attributed the findings to auditory distraction and/or increased emotional arousal that diverts cognitive capacity. Negative interpersonal interactions seem to exert multiple negative effects: disrupting case flow (inefficiency), distracting other team members (who witness the interaction), and decreasing team performance in others (by increasing stress and decreasing psychological safety).

Prevention/Mitigation

Education in multitasking, distraction management, and stress coping strategies is helpful, especially for trainees and junior staff.[47,64] Health care providers are notoriously poor at taking the same advice they give patients. Providers should be encouraged to get adequate sleep, regular exercise, adhere to sound ergonomic principles during surgery, and maintain adequate nutrition and hydration (even on busy OR days). Such self-care is at odds with traditional surgical culture, which greatly values heroics and self-sacrifice whatever the personal cost. However, as in high-performance athletics, peak physical condition can maximize intraoperative psychomotor and cognitive performance and increase one's ability to manage the inevitable interruptions and distractions of the OR. Barriers to reducing negative distractions and interruptions include resistance to change surgical processes, ingrained surgical culture, and providers' poor understanding of the negative performance impact of distractions. However, elimination of unnecessary distractions is a crucial step in maximizing the quality and efficiency of the surgical care provided.

HOW THE ACOUSTIC SPACE AFFECTS CONCENTRATION, PATIENT CARE, AND WORKFLOW
Acoustic Space

The acoustic space is defined as the interaction between sound and a room and has important effects on clinical workflow and patient care.[65] Electronic and mechanical sources of noise pollution can interfere with clinical duties requiring cognition and concentration,[48,66] and essential team communication is impaired by poor speech discrimination, sound reverberation, and background noise, including music.[67] These impairments in mental efficiency, short-term memory, and communication not only limit clinical efficiency, but can have serious consequences for the patient.[66] Modulating and improving the clinical acoustic space can improve workflow and patient safety.

Noise

To prevent hearing loss, the National Institute for Occupational Safety and Health Agency recommends a limit of 85 dB for an 8-hour exposure period and a limit of 100 dB for a 15-minute period.[48] Common sources of hospital noise are alarms (60–85 dB), fans (60–85 dB), vacuum aspiration systems (50–60 dB), conversations (70–80 dB), and background music (80–90 dB).[65]

In such areas as the OR, walls and other parallel flat surfaces are impervious to water and increase noise by reflecting sound.[65] During neurosurgical and orthopedic procedures, noise exceeds 100 dB more than 40% of the time, levels comparable with a busy freeway, and can reach 130 dB.[48] Rather than being a quiet and calm environment, the noise in the OR resembles a loud busy restaurant[68] and can interfere with safe and efficient patient care.[48,66] The detrimental effects of noise on intraoperative clinical care requiring psychomotor tasks, attention, memory, auditory processing, and communication[66,69] have led to independent position statements on noise and distraction from the Association of Perioperative Nurses,[70] American College of Surgeons,[71] and American Society of Anesthesiologists.[72]

Intraoperative Music: Effects on Clinical Workflow

A unique form of sound, music is an integral part of surgery today[73] and an important component of the acoustic space with its own effects on clinical workflow, communication, and patient care.[67,74,75] For surgeons, music has been shown to reduce stress and improve the speed and quality of surgical closures.[76,77] However, in one survey more than 50% of anesthesiologists believe music is a distraction if a patient is having anesthetic-related problems.[74] The distracting effect is even higher for music the anesthesiologist does not like[48] and, in some instances, music can mask intraoperative alarms.[78]

Intraoperative music can affect workflow by impairing communication among OR staff.[67,79] In 2015 Weldon and coworkers[67] videotaped 20 operations and demonstrated that music in the OR resulted in requests from surgeons to nurses being repeated five times more often compared with when music was not played. The signal-to-noise ratio for effective communication requires that speech be 10 dB higher than background noise, but because surgical masks preclude lip-reading, this ratio is higher in the OR.[80] Additionally, sound reverberation impairs speech discrimination, and the auditory processing function of surgeons worsens in the presence of background music.[79] In Weldon's study, it was observed that "Sometimes it took a while to reduce the volume on the sound system, for instance, when a nurse was trying to find the volume control on an anesthetist's iPod. Such delays in minimizing noise and rapid changes in volume can become critical for safety, especially during emergencies when hearing and speaking clearly are paramount."[67]

Optimizing the control of intraoperative music volume has the potential to improve workflow and patient safety. Placing a volume controller close to the anesthesiologist allows music to be manually muted at important times, such as sterile communication periods, and can be done when the circulating room nurse is engaged in other tasks. An additional improvement is the adoption of a "smart" music volume controller that is integrated with the patient's intraoperative vital signs.[81] Intelligent integration of the OR music system is technically feasible[81,82] and may be considered as part of a comprehensive strategy to minimize noise and distraction.[70] Opportunities exist to improve the acoustic space through reductions of overall noise, improvements in acoustics, and advancements in alarm and music technology. As health care systems strive to become high-reliability organizations (eg, nuclear and aviation), optimizing the acoustic space can lead to improvements in workflow and patient safety.

CLINICAL WORKFLOW: TECHNIQUES FOR THE INTENSIVE CARE UNIT

A recent overall increase in patient acuity has presented unique challenges for the critical care physician.[83] Zimmerman and colleagues[83] describe that the mean Acute Physiology Score and the number of patients with more than one chronic health condition have increased in the last 25 years, and a Swedish research group found that critically ill patients were sicker and required more time-intensive care.[84] At the same time, hospital length of stay is shortened as hospitals re-engineer clinical workflow. Several propositions have been made to improve clinical workflow and ensure high-quality care for critically ill patients.

Multidisciplinary Rounds

A multidisciplinary team is a patient-centered model of care wherein all stakeholders involved in a patient's care, including the patient and the patient's family, come together in a concerted effort to make decisions for the well-being of the patient. There are a variety of rounding models, including teaching rounds, safety rounds, stewardship rounds, transitions of care rounds, and rounds that focus on patient discharge from the hospital. The multidisciplinary ICU team may include, but is not limited to, physicians, nurses, pharmacists, respiratory therapists, physical therapists, dieticians, social workers, chaplains, and hospital administrators. Some rounding models may include individuals to assist with billing and coding and quality improvement and hospital utilization management. Each discipline brings a unique knowledge base and skill set, and each can contribute to improving overall outcomes for the patient.

Team rounding on every patient every day allows each clinical expert to discuss the patient in real time, maximizing efficiency; improving communication between health care providers; and enhancing quality, safety, and the patient experience. Involving the patient and his or her family in the decision-making process also empowers the patient to be invested in their own health care. Multidisciplinary rounds increase the patient care team's understanding of daily goals of care (>85% increase in the number of nurses and medical residents understanding daily goals), decrease ICU length of stay,[85] reduce ventilator days, decrease central line days, improve patient flow through levels of care, and expedite discharge planning.[86] A recent study found that multidisciplinary rounds combined with implementation of bundles, flow meetings for timely decisions and prioritization of activity, and a change in culture to a team-based approach significantly reduced ventilator-associated pneumonias and central line infections. The average ICU length of stay decreased, and a 21% reduction in cost per ICU episode (defined as cost per workload unit $\times$ average length of stay) was noted; no decline in ICU mortality was seen.[87]

In contrast, a 2010 multicenter study (112 hospitals and 107,324 patients) demonstrated that daily multidisciplinary rounds were independently associated with lower ICU mortality. This difference was observed whether low-intensity physician staffing ($P = .01$, defined as optional intensivist consultation or no intensivist) or high-intensity physician staffing ($P<.01$, defined as mandatory consultation or primary intensivist management) was in place. These improved outcomes were attributed to improved implementation of best clinical practices and evidence-based care bundles, reduced adverse drug events, and improved communication between health care providers.[88]

Attention Attrition During Rounds and the Handover Process

Attention attrition during rounds or handovers has been identified as a potential risk factor for patient safety. In the critical care unit, teams and providers routinely take care of more than 10 patients[89] and rounding time in a study by Brown and colleagues[90] was an average 188 minutes per day. With longer rounding and handovers times, an unequal time allotment among different patients has been noted. This phenomenon has been described as "end of round time compression" or "portfolio problem."[91,92] Cohen and coworkers[92] describe that during ICU attending handovers the first patient to be discussed received around 50% more time than the last patient discussed in the same session regardless of severity of illness. By disproportionally allocating time on earlier patients independent of severity of illness, health care providers may potentially increase the risk of decision-making and communication failure with negative effects on patient safety and clinical outcomes. At the same time, the reduction in time spent on later patients might be a surrogate for attention attrition during the rounding or handover process.

There is a paucity of literature addressing alterations to the rounding structure itself. One proposed solution involves the alignment of most time spent per patient with severity of illness. This is achieved by changing the rounding order from the traditional rounding by bed number to rounding by severity of illness. Severity of illness can be determined by scores, such as Sequential Organ Failure Assessment or Acute Physiology and Chronic Health Evaluation.[93] By rethinking clinical workflow, sicker patients are seen earlier during rounds and the "end of round time compression" effect should have less of an effect on patient care and safety.

Telemedicine Intensive Care Unit

The intensivist physician is the leader of the multidisciplinary team and is ultimately responsible for ensuring that clinical care is provided through application of evidence-based best practices. However, many small and geographically rural hospitals lack access to intensivist monitoring of ICU patients. To improve quality of care, at least 40 health care systems in the United States have implemented telemedicine ICUs (tele-ICUs) to help alleviate the shortage of clinically trained intensivist physicians.[94] Tele-ICU allows physicians and nurse intensivists in a centralized or remotely based location to monitor telemetry, vital signs, laboratory data, and electronic health records and provide clinical recommendations to the bedside staff through real-time video conferencing. Implementation of 24-hour tele-ICU in a large academic medical facility with in-house intensivist staffing only during the day (house staff with intensivist telephone case review at night) decreased ICU and hospital mortality, decreased ICU and hospital length of stay, improved adherence to best practices, decreased rates of catheter-related bloodstream infections and ventilator-associated pneumonia, and improved response to alarms for physiologic instability.[95] However, these results have not been consistent among all tele-ICU studies[96,97] and the costs of implementation are substantial (first year implementation costs of $50,000–$100,000 per monitored ICU bed). Associated costs depend on the existing infrastructure of the facility, but can include costs to purchase, install, and maintain the necessary technology; staffing; real estate/property; and other hospital variables, such as nursing supplies and other services (eg, pharmacy, laboratory, radiology).[94]

Although tele-ICU is a viable and attractive option for many facilities, more evidence is needed to fully understand the total impact on patient care. For the facility lacking full-time intensivist support, tele-ICU would theoretically provide an improved level of patient monitoring and care. However, for the hospital that is expanding its ICU presence to other systems through the provision of tele-ICU monitoring, it is impera-tive to remain mindful of the allocation of resources and ensure that patient care at the home institution is not sacrificed.

Building a multidisciplinary team that affords attention to the patient in person and potentially with remote monitoring can improve workflow and communication and potentially attenuate morbidity and improve patient safety.

SUMMARY

The concept of clinical workflow borrows from management and leadership princi-ples outside of medicine. Although medicine is classically compared with aviation, the approach to hierarchy, workflow, and efficiency can be borrowed from business practices. As those principles percolate to medicine, neuroscience is at the root of how clinicians interact with their environment. The only way to rethink clinical work-flow is to understand the neuroscience principles that underlie attention and vigilance. Despite best efforts, internal and external distractors persevere, and without mitigation, no rethinking approach to clinical workflow will be successfully implemented. With any implementation to improve practice, there are human factors that can promote or impede progress. This is especially true in the ICU with many different care providers communicating about the depth and breadth of patients. In that cognitively demanding environment, the multisensory environment (sights and sounds) bombard one with information. Understanding neuroscience aligned with music perception and cognition helps clinicians triage information and provide quality patient care. The most pervasive of these sensory modalities is the auditory stream. Managing the impact of the sound exposure level has impact on patients and clinicians alike. Modulating the environment and working as a team to take care of patients is paramount. However, clinicians must continually rethink clinical workflow, evaluate progress, and understand that other industries have something to offer. When clinicians realize that, they can implement novel approaches and evolve to take the best care of patients—every patient, every time.

REFERENCES

1. Gibbs C. Getting the whole story: reporting and writing the news. New York: Guilford Press; 2003.
2. Imai M. Kaizen, the key to Japan's competitive success. Singapore: McGraw-Hill; 1991.
3. Deming W. The essential Deming: leadership principles from the father of quality. New York: McGraw-Hill; 2013.
4. Pyzdek T. The six sigma handbook: a complete guide to greenbelts, blackbelts, and managers at all levels. Whitehouse Station (NJ): McGraw-Hill; 2001.
5. Cima RR, Brown MJ, Hebl JR, et al. Use of lean and six sigma methodology to improve operating room efficiency in a high-volume tertiary-care academic med-ical center. J Am Coll Surgeons 2011;213(1):83–92.
6. Wood D. Lean and six sigma deployments in hospitals. Am Soc Qual 2009;2(1-4): 13–27.
7. Schneider B. The Oxford handbook of organizational climate and culture. Oxford, United Kingdom: Oxford University Press; 2014.
8. Institute of Medicine Committee on Quality of Health Care in America. In: Kohn LT, Corrigan JM, Donaldson MS, editors. To err is human: building a safer health sys-tem. Washington, DC: National Academies Press (US); 2000. Copyright 2000 by the National Academy of Sciences. All rights reserved.

9. Holden RJ, Carayon P, Gurses AP, et al. SEIPS 2.0: a human factors framework for studying and improving the work of healthcare professionals and patients. Ergonomics 2013;56(11):1669–86.

10. Carayon P, Schoofs Hundt A, Karsh BT, et al. Work system design for patient safety: the SEIPS model. Qual Saf Health Care 2006;15(Suppl 1):i50–8.

11. Donabedian A. The quality of medical care. Science 1978;200(4344):856–64.

12. Mondor TA, Finley GA. The perceived urgency of auditory warning alarms used in the hospital operating room is inappropriate. Can J Anaesth 2003;50(3):221–8.

13. Lukasewicz CL, Mattox EA. Understanding clinical alarm safety. Crit Care Nurse 2015;35(4):45–57.

14. Schmid F, Goepfert MS, Reuter DA. Patient monitoring alarms in the ICU and in the operating room. Crit Care 2013;17(2):216.

15. Borowski M, Görges M, Fried R, et al. Medical device alarms. Biomed Tech (Berl) 2011;56(2):73–83.

16. Graham KC, Cvach M. Monitor alarm fatigue: standardizing use of physiological monitors and decreasing nuisance alarms. Am J Crit Care 2010;19(1):28–34 [quiz: 35].

17. Joint Commission. Medical device alarm safety in hospitals. Sentinel Event Alert 2013;(50):1–3.

18. Rivera-Rodriguez AJ, Karsh BT. Interruptions and distractions in healthcare: review and reappraisal. Qual Saf Health Care 2010;19(4):304–12.

19. Feil M. Distractions and their impact on patient safety. Pa Patient Saf Advis 2013; 10:1–10.

20. Salinas E, Scerra VE, Hauser CK, et al. Decoupling speed and accuracy in an urgent decision-making task reveals multiple contributions to their trade-off. Front Neurosci 2014;8:85.

21. Gladwell M. Outliers. New York: Little, Brown and Company; 2008.

22. Edworthy J, Loxley S, Dennis I. Improving auditory warning design: relationship between warning sound parameters and perceived urgency. Hum Factors 1991;33(2):205–31.

23. Dictionary RHKWsC. Music. 2010; Available at: http://www.kdictionaries-online.com/DictionaryPage.aspx?ApplicationCode=18&DictionaryEntry=music&SearchMode=Entry&TranLangs=18. Accessed 25 March, 2017.

24. Language TAHDotE. Music. 2017; 5th edition: Available at: https://ahdictionary.com/word/search.html?q=music. Accessed 25 March, 2017.

25. Douek J. Music and emotion: a composer's perspective. Front Syst Neurosci 2013;7:82.

26. Harriss EC, editor. Johann Mattheson's Der vollkommene capellmeister: a revised translation with critical commentary. Ann Arbor (MI): UMI Research Press; 1981. No. Studies in Musicology, no. 21.

27. Sanderson PM, Wee A, Lacherez P. Learnability and discriminability of melodic medical equipment alarms. Anaesthesia 2006;61(2):142–7.

28. Chrysomallis M. Dies irae in the soundtrack of horror. 2016; Available at: https://www.primephonic.com/news-dies-irae-in-the-soundtrack-of-horror. Accessed 26 March, 2017.

29. Gregory R. Dies irae. Music Lett 1953;34(2):113–39.

30. Ploger M. 2017.

31. Lucas G, Hamill M, Ford H, et al. Star wars. Episode IV, A new hope. New hope. In: Enhanced trilogy version. ed. Beverly Hills (CA): 20th Century Fox Home Entertainment; 2006.

32. Bribitzer-Stull M. Understanding the leitmotif: from Wagner to Hollywood film music. Cambridge (United Kingdom): Cambridge University Press; 2015.
33. IEC. International Standard 60601-1-8 (2005): Medical electrical equipment- part 1-8: general requirements for safety- collateral standard. General requirements, tests and guidance for alarm systems in medical electrical equipment and medical electrical systems. Geneva (Switzerland): International Electrotechnical Commission; 2005.
34. Wee AN, Sanderson PM. Are melodic medical equipment alarms easily learned? Anesth Analg 2008;106(2):501–8. Table of contents.
35. Edworthy J, Hellier E. Alarms and human behaviour: implications for medical alarms. Br J Anaesth 2006;97(1):12–7.
36. Lacherez P, Seah EL, Sanderson P. Overlapping melodic alarms are almost indiscriminable. Hum Factors 2007;49(4):637–45.
37. Gillard J, Schutz M. Composing alarms: considering the musical aspects of auditory alarm design. Neurocase 2016;22(6):566–76.
38. Daunizeau J, den Ouden HEM, Pessiglione M, et al. Observing the observer (I): meta-Bayesian models of learning and decision-making. PLoS One 2010;5:e15554.
39. Posner MI. Orienting of attention. J Exp Psychol 1980;32:3–25.
40. Kanwisher N, Wojciulik E. Visual attention: insights from brain imaging. Nat Rev Neurosci 2000;1:91–100.
41. Desimone R, Duncan J. Neural mechanisms of selective visual attention. Annu Rev Neurosci 1995;18:193–222.
42. Wu CT, Weissman DH, Roberts KC, et al. The neural circuitry underlying the executive control of auditory spatial attention. Brain Res 2007;1134:187–98.
43. Smith DV, Davis B, Niu K, et al. Spatial attention evokes similar activation patterns for visual and auditory stimuli. J Cogn Neurosci 2010;22:347–61.
44. Allen K, Alais D, Carlile S. Speech intelligibility reduces over distance from an attended location: evidence for an auditory spatial gradient of attention. Atten Percept Psychophys 2009;71:164–73.
45. Spagna A, Mackie MA, Fan J. Supramodal executive control of attention. Front Psychol 2015;6:65.
46. Bregman AS. Auditory scene analysis: the perceptual organization of sound. Cambridge (MA): The MIT Press; 1990. p. 773.
47. Mentis HM, Chellali A, Manser K, et al. A systematic review of the effect of distraction on surgeon performance: directions for operating room policy and surgical training. Surg Endosc 2016;30(5):1713–24.
48. Katz JD. Noise in the operating room. Anesthesiology 2014;121(4):894–8.
49. Yoong W, Khin A, Ramlal N, et al. Interruptions and distractions in the gynaecological operating theatre: irritating or dangerous? Ergonomics 2015;58(8):1314–9.
50. Pluyter JR, Buzink SN, Rutkowski AF, et al. Do absorption and realistic distraction influence performance of component task surgical procedure? Surg Endosc 2010;24(4):902–7.
51. Persoon MC, van Putten K, Muijtjens AM, et al. Effect of distraction on the performance of endourological tasks: a randomized controlled trial. BJU Int 2011;107(10):1653–7.
52. Sevdalis N, Undre S, McDermott J, et al. Impact of intraoperative distractions on patient safety: a prospective descriptive study using validated instruments. World J Surg 2014;38(4):751–8.
53. Wiegmann DA, ElBardissi AW, Dearani JA, et al. Disruptions in surgical flow and their relationship to surgical errors: an exploratory investigation. Surgery 2007;142(5):658–65.

54. Wong DR, Torchiana DF, Vander Salm TJ, et al. Impact of cardiac intraoperative precursor events on adverse outcomes. Surgery 2007;141(6):715–22.

55. Jothiraj H, Howland-Harris J, Evley R, et al. Distractions and the anaesthetist: a qualitative study of context and direction of distraction. Br J Anaesth 2013; 111(3):477–82.

56. Wetzel CM, Kneebone RL, Woloshynowych M, et al. The effects of stress on surgical performance. Am J Surg 2006;191(1):5–10.

57. Dabholkar T, Yardi S, Dabholkar Y. Prevalence of work-related musculoskeletal symptoms in surgeons performing minimally invasive surgery: a review of literature. Int Surg J 2016;3(3):1028–34.

58. Driskell JE, Salas E. Stress and human performance. Mahwah (NJ): Lawrence Erlbaum Associates; 1996.

59. Eysenck MW, Calvo MG. Anxiety and performance: the processing efficiency theory. Cogn Emot 1992;6(6):409–34.

60. Rogers D, Lingard L, Boehler ML, et al. Teaching operating room conflict management to surgeons: clarifying the optimal approach. Med Educ 2011;45(9): 939–45.

61. Rosenstein AH, O'Daniel M. Impact and implications of disruptive behavior in the perioperative arena. J Am Coll Surgeons 2006;203(1):96–105.

62. Flin R, Yule S, McKenzie L, et al. Attitudes to teamwork and safety in the operating theatre. Surgeon 2006;4(3):145–51.

63. Riskin A, Erez A, Foulk TA, et al. The impact of rudeness on medical team performance: a randomized trial. Pediatrics 2015;136(3):487–95.

64. Bongers PJ, Diederick van Hove P, Stassen LP, et al. A new virtual-reality training module for laparoscopic surgical skills and equipment handling: can multitasking be trained? a randomized controlled trial. J Surg Educ 2015;72(2):184–91.

65. Oliveira CR, Arenas GW. Occupational exposure to noise pollution in anesthesiology. Rev Bras Anestesiol 2012;62(2):253–61.

66. Murthy VS, Malhotra SK, Bala I, et al. Detrimental effects of noise on anaesthetists. Can J Anaesth 1995;42(7):608–11.

67. Weldon SM, Korkiakangas T, Bezemer J, et al. Music and communication in the operating theatre. J Adv Nurs 2015;71(12):2763–74.

68. Smith-Strickland K. Should doctors be allowed to listen to music during surgery? 2015; online article. Available at: http://gizmodo.com/rockin-in-the-or-the-debate-over-music-in-surgery-1742431576. Accessed November 13, 2015.

69. Stevenson RA, Schlesinger JJ, Wallace MT. Effects of divided attention and operating room noise on perception of pulse oximeter pitch changes: a laboratory study. Anesthesiology 2013;118(2):376–81.

70. AORN position statement on managing distractions and noise during perioperative patient care. AORN J 2014;99(1):22–6.

71. American College of Surgeons. Statement on distractions in the operating room. 2016; ACS website. Available at: www.facs.org/about~acs/statements/89-distractions. Accessed October 1, 2016.

72. American Society of Anesthesiologists. American Society of Anesthesiologists Committee on Quality Management and Departmental Administration (QMDA). Statement on distractions. 2016; ASA website. Available at: www.asahq.org/~/media/Sites/ASAHQ/Files/Public/Resources/standards-guidelines/statement-on-distractions. Accessed January 27, 2016.

73. Shambo L, Umadhay T, Pedoto A. Music in the operating room: is it a safety hazard? AANA J 2015;83(1):43–8.

74. Strickland RA. Music in the operating room: harmony or discord? Bull Anesth Hist 2007;25(3):10–2.
75. Hawksworth C, Asbury AJ, Millar K. Music in theatre: not so harmonious. A survey of attitudes to music played in the operating theatre. Anaesthesia 1997;52(1): 79–83.
76. Lies SR, Zhang AY. Prospective randomized study of the effect of music on the efficiency of surgical closures. Aesthet Surg J 2015;35(7):858–63.
77. Allen K, Blascovich J. Effects of music on cardiovascular reactivity among surgeons. JAMA 1994;272(11):882–4.
78. Anesthesia Patient Safety Foundation. A case report from the anesthesia incident reporting system. ASA Monitor 2016;6:36–7.
79. Way TJ, Long A, Weihing J, et al. Effect of noise on auditory processing in the operating room. J Am Coll Surg 2013;216(5):933–8.
80. Ross LA, Saint-Amour D, Leavitt VM, et al. Do you see what I am saying? Exploring visual enhancement of speech comprehension in noisy environments. Cereb Cortex 2007;17(5):1147–53.
81. MacDonald A. Smart operating room music. Anesth Analgesia 2015;121(3):836.
82. Schlesinger JJ. In response. Anesth Analg 2015;121(3):836.
83. Zimmerman JE, Kramer AA, Knaus WA. Changes in hospital mortality for United States intensive care unit admissions from 1988 to 2012. Crit Care 2013;17(2):R81.
84. Levenstam AK, Bergbom I. Changes in patients' need of nursing care reflected in the Zebra system. J Nurs Management 2002;10(4):191–9.
85. Pronovost P, Berenholtz S, Dorman T, et al. Improving communication in the ICU using daily goals. J Crit Care 2003;18(2):71–5.
86. Improvement Map: Getting started kit: multidiscipinary rounds how-to guide. Institute for healthcare improvement. 2010.
87. Jain M, Miller L, Belt D, et al. Decline in ICU adverse events, nosocomial infections and cost through a quality improvement initiative focusing on teamwork and culture change. Qual Saf Health Care 2006;15(4):235–9.
88. Kim MM, Barnato AE, Angus DC, et al. The effect of multidisciplinary care teams on intensive care unit mortality. Arch Intern Med 2010;170(4):369–76.
89. Groeger JS, Strosberg MA, Halpern NA, et al. Descriptive analysis of critical care units in the United States. Crit Care Med 1992;20(6):846–63.
90. Brown SES, Rey MM, Pardo D, et al. The allocation of intensivists' rounding time under conditions of intensive care unit capacity strain. Am J Respir Crit Care Med 2014;190(7):831–4.
91. Kannampallil T, Jones L, Buchman T, et al. 638: last patients finish last: end of round time compression during CT ICU clinical rounds. Crit Care Med 2011; 39(12):176.
92. Cohen MD, Ilan R, Garrett L, et al. The earlier the longer: disproportionate time allocated to patients discussed early in attending physician handoff sessions. Arch Intern Med 2012;172(22):1762–4.
93. Knaus WA, Draper EA, Wagner DP, et al. APACHE II: a severity of disease classification system. Crit Care Med 1985;13(10):818–29.
94. Kumar G, Falk DM, Bonello RS, et al. The costs of critical care telemedicine programs: a systematic review and analysis. Chest 2013;143(1):19–29.
95. Lilly CM, Cody S, Zhao H, et al. Hospital mortality, length of stay, and preventable complications among critically ill patients before and after tele-ICU reengineering of critical care processes. JAMA 2011;305(21):2175–83.

96. Thomas EJ, Lucke JF, Wueste L, et al. Association of telemedicine for remote monitoring of intensive care patients with mortality, complications, and length of stay. JAMA 2009;302(24):2671–8.

97. Young LB, Chan PS, Lu X, et al. Impact of telemedicine intensive care unit coverage on patient outcomes: a systematic review and meta-analysis. Arch Intern Med 2011;171(6):498–506.

Developing Capacity to Do Improvement Science Work

Irene McGhee, MD, FRCP[a],*, Yehoshua Gleicher, MSc, MD, FRCP[b]

KEYWORDS

- Capacity building • Co-learning • Behavior change • Influence
- Stakeholder engagement • Perioperative care transitions

KEY POINTS

- Quality improvement efforts require the collaboration of patients, providers, and leadership.
- Creating co-learning opportunities that are interprofessional translates to more effective improvement capacity at the bedside.
- Behavior change is complex. Anticipating and planning strategies based on motivation, opportunity, and capability can be useful.

INTRODUCTION

An important feature of learning health care systems is that they measure performance and strive to attain and maintain high-quality care using quality improvement (QI) principles. Hardwiring QI into health care systems to make them learn requires at least 4 factors. First, visionary leadership is needed to provide direction aligned with organizational objectives and to provide resources to support QI efforts. Second, adequate training in QI and related disciplines is needed at all levels of health care organizations, from leadership to frontline staff to support services. Third, those engaged in QI must possess understanding of the factors that drive behavior change as well as each setting's unique needs and work environment. Finally, patients and families should be brought into the QI team as much as possible, and opportunities for learning with and from patients should be sought.

In this article, these factors and challenges are discussed as part of the process of developing capacity to do health system–based improvement work.

All authors put forth a disclosure statement that the work submitted does not have commercial or financial conflicts of interest and no funding sources.

[a] Anesthesiology, Sunnybrook Health Sciences Centre, University of Toronto, 2075 Bayview Avenue, Toronto, Ontario M4N 3M5, Canada; [b] Anesthesiology, Mount Sinai Health Centre, University of Toronto, 600 University Avenue, Toronto, Ontario M5G 1X5, Canada
* Corresponding author.
E-mail address: Irene.mcghee@sunnybrook.ca

DEFINITION

In this article, *developing capacity* is defined as the development of processes that facilitate the conduct of health care improvement work at a health system level. The scope of developing capacity is explained by Batalden and Davidoff in their definition of QI work: "...the combined and unceasing efforts of everyone—healthcare professionals, patients and their families, researchers, payers, planners and educators—to make changes that will lead to better patient outcomes (health), better system performance (care) and better professional development."[1] It follows that developing capacity is an active process involving many—from individuals to organizations to systems. In summary, developing capacity building starts with raising awareness and understanding of the scope and complexity of QI and addressing the enablers and barriers to the integration of QI into health care systems: leadership, training, applying QI principles, and partnering with patients and families to do improvement work.

LEADERSHIP: LEADING CHANGE

Leadership is not about making clever decisions or doing bigger deals, it is about helping release the positive energy that exists naturally within people...
                                                                              —Henry Mintzberg

The sobering reality is that concepts do not just transform into practice. Understanding the importance of QI and believing in the ability of health systems to change is insufficient to create and sustain a mature, productive, and impactful QI program. That said, leadership is a necessary first step to supporting an organizational culture that embraces QI. Leaders also control the resources necessary to execute QI efforts. Leading change is the enabling competency necessary to build capacity.

John Kotter has written several books about organizational change management, books acknowledging that change is anathema to the human condition. His and Rathgeber's lighthearted book, *Our Iceberg is Melting*,[2] demonstrates the principles behind leading change by telling the story of a group of penguins dealing with a changing world. Specifically, he deals with the complexities of managing teams with diverse interests, all of whom seem hardwired to resist change.

Beyond Kotter and Rathgeber's book, there are important theories that provide insight into the ways that change occurs and the processes through which change diffuses through groups and organizations. A detailed treatment of these theories is beyond the scope of this article, but interested readers are referred to Prochaskas and DiClemente's[3] Transtheoretical Model of Change (which includes precontemplation, contemplation, preparation, action, and maintenance) and Rogers'[4] *Diffusion of Innovations*.

From the authors' perspective, capacity building—getting people on board—starts with fostering connections through meaningful conversations with stakeholders, which helps develop relationships that form the foundation for influence and leadership. Grenny[5] describes the importance of organizational influence and sets out a framework defining the various opportunities necessary, partnered with ability and motivation factors, to lead change successfully.

The authors offer the following example to illustrate key leadership principles that apply to creating change in organizations, which include understanding motivation:

- You notice "x" (and you think "x" is a problem).
- You show interest in "x" — why is "x" a problem, and for whom is it a problem?

- You listen to a broad cross-section of stakeholders, including leaders, frontline providers, and others, to discover how "x" became the status quo.
- You try to understand the motivation driving "x," before deciding "y" or "z" is the solution.
- You demonstrate curiosity, exploring the situation and striving for understanding.
- You work with a team to create solutions collaboratively to increase the likelihood of sustainable change.

Another reference that lays out key principles for communicating and collaborating effectively when faced with challenge and change is *Thanks for the Feedback* by Stone and Heen.[6] This book goes far beyond feedback—it promotes self-reflection and learning that can enable leading change that is more pull focused than push focused.

Effective leadership that promotes commitment to a common purpose is just the first step to developing capacity to do improvement work. A second vital factor is training in QI.

TRAINING AND CREATING COMMON PURPOSE

Meaningful QI activities require the application of knowledge of QI principles and related concepts. From an educational perspective, application of knowledge is a higher-order cognitive function than simply possessing knowledge. According to Miller's[7] triangle, steps along the continuum of knowledge include the following: knows, knows how, shows how/applies, and does. To develop competency at the higher "applies" level, educational curricula for health professionals should be designed to provide both grounding in the basic principles of QI (knows) and QI methodologies (knows how).

There are numerous sources to guide the development and delivery of QI curricula. Examples of these include the Institute for Healthcare Improvement,[8] the Canadian Patient Safety Institute Patient Safety Education Program,[9] the Advancing Safety for Patients in Residency Education[10] initiative, the Health Foundation,[11] and the World Health Organization Patient Safety Curriculum Guide for Medical Schools.[12] Regardless of the approach chosen, educational goals and objectives should be selected that meet the needs of the organization and the needs of the learners. Instructional design and teaching methods should incorporate cognitive, psychomotor, and affective domains. This is best supported by providing opportunity for active discussion and interaction among learners with an experienced facilitator and reviewing evidence from various sources and discussing different perspectives. Given that QI is, by its nature, a multidisciplinary activity, opportunities to integrate learner types should be sought.

Once learners possess basic QI knowledge and skills (knowing and knowing how), a shared awareness is created that can serve as a springboard for application of this knowledge to QI efforts by trainees, coworkers, faculty, and other health professionals in their workplaces. Keeping these stakeholders engaged and facilitating their collaboration is key for success, at the system, organization, and individual levels.

After training, the work of developing capacity continues by creating a sense of common purpose. In the literature, key concepts have been identified that relate to this purpose, concepts that operate at the system/organizational level and at the individual level.

At the system level, ideally, QI is set out as a priority in an institution's charter (mission, vision, and values) and is championed by its leaders (see "Leading Change," discussed previously). QI should be seen as an integral part of daily clinical work. Efforts should be made to engage patients and families in this work and health professional students and their teachers in participating as co-learners in QI training initiatives. Assessment of this system-wide QI work is tracked by developing metrics focusing on the patient, team, and system levels.[13–16]

At the individual level, QI work must be perceived as real and relevant to clinical practice. Adults learn best when they have a personal need to know. For this reason, a good starting point is a needs assessment to identify gaps between an individual's current practice and best practice. This can create a sense of urgency for change and provide ideas for projects to improve care quality.

Promoting active engagement with local experts and encouraging participation in QI projects already under way lead to application of learning to a learner's own work environment. Robust follow-up and feedback systems, including mentorship, role-modeling, networking opportunities, co-learning, and ongoing training, help maintain momentum and can support spread and sustainability.[17–20]

Although training in QI principles and methodologies is important, knowledge acquisition, per se, does not lead to the organizational behavior change needed to improve care quality. Behavior change is itself complex, but there are theories that provide some insight into how to achieve durable behavior change.

UNDERSTANDING BEHAVIORAL CHANGE

Just telling people to change and do "y" instead of "x" does not work. Rather, successful behavior change requires alignment of many factors. Knoster[21,22] details the management of complex change, discussing 5 factors involved in change—vision, skills, incentives, resources, and an action plan. They also discusses the disruptive consequences when any one of these factors is missing (**Fig. 1**). Understanding, anticipating, and planning ahead can avoid these disruptions, which can be difficult to reverse once present.

An additional factor to consider in changing behavior is that there are individual differences in how situations are perceived and how thinking about problems is approached. de Bono's book—*The 6 Thinking Hats*[23] is a great primer on exploring the various perspectives of any issue and the importance of being ready to address various perspectives in 6 different ways to find the best approach in a given context (**Fig. 2**).

An alternative way of thinking about behavior change is advanced by the Behavior Change Wheel theory (**Fig. 3**).[24,25] It is grounded in context and asks, What factors in the present population at the present time underlie variation in the behavioral parameter?

According to the Behavior Change Wheel, there are 3 areas to target when considering behavior change. These 3 areas are illustrated using the example of appropriate and effective handwashing behavior:

1. Motivation: Motivation can be intrinsic—"I want to wash my hands well because it is the right thing to do for my patients" —and/or, extrinsic—"my infection rate statistics have not been great lately" or perhaps "someone with administrative clout is watching how well I wash my hands."
2. Opportunity: Opportunity is about how easy it is to do the right thing. An example of opportunity is ensuring that there are many handwashing dispensers in convenient locations everywhere or that the dispensers that are present are always kept full and functioning properly.
3. Capability: Capability characterizes the ability of an actor to execute a desired behavior. In the handwashing example, capability is achieved by ensuring that people know how to wash their hands appropriately.

Conditions for Successful Implementation

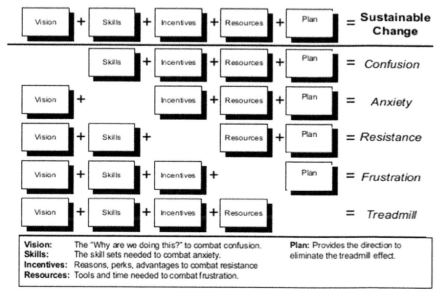

Fig. 1. Managing complex change. (*From* Knoster T, Villa R, Thousand J. A framework for thinking about systems change. In: Villa R, Thousand J, editors. Restructuring for caring and effective education: Piecing the puzzle together. Baltimore (MD): Paul H. Brookes Publishing Co; 2000; with permission.)

Edward de Bono's Six Thinking Hats Model for Critical Thinking and Problem Solving

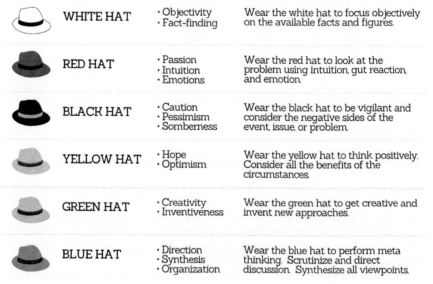

Fig. 2. Six thinking hats. (*From* Goodman E. The effective team's high performance workbook. RiverRhee Publishing; 2014; with permission.)

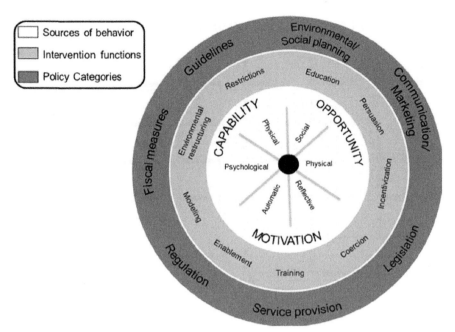

Fig. 3. Behavior change wheel. (*Modified from* Michies S, van Stralen MM, West R. The behaviour change wheel: a new method for characterising and designing behaviour change interventions. Implement Sci 2011;6(42); with permission.)

The handwashing example greatly simplifies the actual Behavior Change Wheel theory. Each of the 3 areas—motivation, opportunity and capability—can be further broken down and more comprehensive strategies developed, as required by a given situation.[25] Eid and Quinn[26] analysis revealed that trainee characteristics, their work environment, and the training course were most influential for assuring transfer of training. The successful transfer of training could be seen to align with the 3 areas set out in the Behavior Change Wheel. Individual trainees' motivation (trainee characteristic), their opportunity (work environment), and their capability (the training course they received) were key predictors of behavioral change (successful training transfer).

Understanding the theory of behavior change is instrumental to devising strategies to enable successful implementation of improvement activities in health care. The next step to developing capacity to doing QI work is to get people started in the application of QI knowledge and behavior change principles.

APPLYING QUALITY IMPROVEMENT KNOWLEDGE: PRACTICAL STRATEGIES

The people around you, your peers and coworkers, are the best assets to building capacity. Start with where they are and ask what matters to them. Everyone in the health care system has ideas about quality and how to improve it. An important first step is to ask yourself, Is the problem identified based on your view of the world or is it shared by others? Conducting an opinion survey of the problem helps answer this question and better understand what others see and think.

Working effectively toward a common goal requires an inclusive approach. Follow this up with a survey asking for illustrative examples and stories to clarify the various perspectives present in the stakeholders. This makes a project real and relevant.

Marshall Ganz[27,28] states, "every change idea needs a narrative/STORY (lead with the 'heart'), a STRATEGY (a plan for how it *could* work—the 'brain') and an ACTION plan." What is needed to execute the plan?

Start with the development of an AIM statement that is specific—how much and by when? (As articulated by Don Berwick, "Some is not a number, and soon is not a time.")[29]

Process mapping, root cause analysis, and other brainstorming activities can improve everyone's understanding of the issues and inform strategy.

The measurement and collection of real time data, for example, dashboards, are instrumental in keeping people focused and motivated. Social media—Twitter, chat-rooms, and blogs—provide platforms for idea sharing and creative collaboration[27] and can keep everyone updated about "where we're at and where we're going." Also, by providing stakeholders with regular feedback that is specific, measurable, attainable, relevant, and timely (SMART), the team is energized and propelled forward toward their shared purpose.

This same energy can be spread by "talking the talk, while walking the walk." Hallway conversations and any interaction with others in an institution (and beyond) can be viewed as an opportunity to build capacity. Crafting an elevator pitch that clearly articulates the problem addressed, the project strategy, and how it aligns with an institution's vision, mission, and values is a powerful tool. As physicians, most do not have a well-developed marketing/promotion skill set.

A project manager/assistant is indispensable to help with this and continually push the agenda, provide support, gather data, anticipate problems, and troubleshoot inevitable setbacks. Engage administration for support and learn how to tap into the QI resources that already exist in the institution. (There is no point in reinventing the wheel or running parallel projects.) Volunteer and engage in local quality committees because this inside track may reveal other opportunities for networking. The process of building social capital is an ongoing process and enables successful current and future project development.

PERIOPERATIVE QUALITY IMPROVEMENT OPPORTUNITIES

The perioperative care period presents unique challenges in growing social capital. This period is marked by multiple transitions of care over short time periods. Such task-focused care encounters are often short on meaningful interactions with co-workers and patients.

Buy-in (stakeholder engagement) takes time. In the real world, production pressure and other conflicting agendas can make this difficult. Perioperative professionals are at a disadvantage when trying to insert into these transitory settings that require iterative processes, even though the ultimate goal is to improve quality.

Viewed another way, however, this challenging setting may present unique QI opportunities. Communication problems are a major factor in adverse events—this is especially germane when the care of patients is frequently changing hands (as in the perioperative period). The perioperative team is perfectly positioned to improve communication across the many transitions of care patient's experience in this setting (eg, developing standardized handovers and checklists). Patients are the only constant in this dynamic complexity.

INCLUDING PATIENTS AND FAMILIES IN QUALITY IMPROVEMENT

Patients must come off the sidelines and onto the pitch. Empowering citizens and patients to help prevent and manage their own conditions, facilitated by new tools

*and technologies, has great potential for improving outcomes and reducing ever-
increasing demand on health systems.*
    —The Global Health Policy Summit Report in 2012, United Kingdom

Patients coming for surgery are highly motivated. The stakes are high and their well-
ness is on the line. For this reason, the perioperative period presents an ideal opportunity to build capacity with patients proactively.

Patients and their families can be drivers of QI initiatives. Their unique perspectives
can inform and guide ways to improving health care (eg, patient-related experiences
and patient-related outcome measures).[30] Although routines may have to shift to
accommodate patients and families, the effort to do so is likely to pay dividends in
the form of QI initiatives that have lasting value for patients. Some institutions have
created patient and family advisory councils to facilitate ongoing conversations about
the ways that health care can better meet patients' needs.

SUMMARY

Building capacity starts with making connections with patients, coworkers, and
others about quality issues that matter to them. Provonost summarized the steps
to QI activities—engage, educate, execute, and evaluate. A how-to guide to QI in
ICUs and an introduction to the checklist concept were transformational to safer patient care.[31]

Providing the best care is our common purpose. Institutions can promote a change-
ready culture; The Human Resources department advises all new hires that the organization is committed to continuous QI, specifically stating that all employees are
expected to do their best work and also to improve on it. Training opportunities are
provided to enable this capability (with an "I-LEAD" program championed by Brigette
Hales (et al) Director, Quality and Patient Safety, SHSC, personal communication,
2016).

What really matters to all of us is best understood by our stories. They teach us
about what is working well and what is working not so well. Stories spark engagement
of both patients and providers. They are the evidence and drivers to ensure care processes are continuously reviewed, revised, and operationalized. Execution of QI initiatives requires an understanding of leading change and the critical contributions of
opportunity, capability, and motivation in behavior change. Ongoing feedback and
evaluation are also essential in complex dynamic systems. Hardwiring these processes creates a transparent, accountable, responsive health care system that is
ready to meet the complex needs of the future.

REFERENCES

1. Batalden PB, Davidoff F. What is "quality improvement" and how can it transform healthcare? Qual Saf Health Care 2007;16(1):2–3.
2. Kotter JP, Rathgeber H. Our iceberg is melting: changing and succeeding under any conditions. New York: St. Martin's Press; 2006.
3. Prochaskas JO, DiClemente CC. Processes of self-change of smoking: toward an integrative model of change. J Consult Clin Psychol 1983;51(3):390–5.
4. Rogers E. Diffusion of innovations. Canada: Simon and Schuster; 2003.
5. Grenny J. Influencer: the new science of leading change. New York: McGraw-Hill; 2013.
6. Stone D, Heen S. Thanks for the feedback: the art and science of receiving feed-back well. New York: Viking; 2014.

7. Miller GE. The assessment of clinical skills/competence/performance. Acad Med 1990;65:63–7.
8. Frankel A, Haraden C, Federico F, et al. A framework for safe, reliable, and effective care. Cambridge (MA): Institute for Healthcare Improvement and Safe & Reliable Healthcare; 2017.
9. Emanuel L, Taylor L, Hain A, et al, editors. The patient safety education program. Ottawa (Canada): CPSI (Canadian Patient Safety Institute) Curriculum; 2011.
10. Advancing Safety for Patients in Residency Education (ASPIRE): 2013, 2015 Royal College of Physicians & Surgeons of Canada and the Canadian Patient Safety Institute, Ottawa, Canada.
11. Evidence scan: quality improvement for healthcare professionals. United Kingdom: The Health Foundation; 2012.
12. Walton M, Woodward H, Van Staalduinen S, et al. The WHO patient safety curriculum guide for medical schools. Qual Saf Health Care 2010;19:542–6.
13. Cooke M, Ironside PM, Ogrinc GS. Mainstreaming quality and safety: a reformulation of quality and safety education for health professions students. BMJ Qual Saf 2011;20(Suppl):1–7.
14. Price D. Continuing medical education, quality improvement, and organizational change: implications of recent theories for twenty-first-century CME. Med Teach 2005;27(3):259–68.
15. Leach DC. Changing education to improve patient care. Qual Health Care 2001; 10(Suppl 2):ii54–8.
16. Ladden MD, Bednash G, Stevens DP, et al. Educating interprofessional learners for quality, safety and systems improvement. J Interprof Care 2006;20(5): 497–505.
17. Patow CA, Karpovich K, Riesenberg LA, et al. Residents' engagement in quality improvement: a systematic review of the literature. Acad Med 2009;84(12): 1757–64.
18. Wong BM, Levinson W, Shojania KG. Quality improvement in medical education: current state and future directions. Med Educ 2012;46(1):107–19.
19. Wong BM, Kuper A, Hollenberg E, et al. Sustaining quality improvement and patient safety training in graduate medical education: lessons from social theory. Acad Med 2013;88(8):1149–56.
20. Wong BM, Etchells EE, Kuper A, et al. Teaching quality improvement and patient safety to trainees: a systematic review. Acad Med 2010;85(9):1425–39.
21. Villa R, Thousand J, editors. Restructuring for caring and effective education: Piecing the puzzle together. Baltimore (MD): Paul H. Brookes Publishing Co; 2000.
22. Available at: http://www.belb.org.uk/downloads/rc_knoster_managing_complex_change.pdf.
23. De Bono E. Six thinking hats. New York: Little Brown & Company; 1985. updated 1999.
24. Michie S, van Stralen MM, West R. The behaviour change wheel: a new method for characterising and designing behaviour change interventions. Implement Sci 2011;6:42.
25. Handley MA, Gorukanti A, Cattamanchi A. Strategies for implementing implementation science: a methodological overview. Emerg Med J 2016;33(9):660–4.
26. Eid A, Quinn D. Factors predicting training transfer in health professionals participating in quality improvement educational interventions. BMC Med Educ 2017; 17(1):26.

27. Available at: http://marshallganz.usmblogs.com/files/2012/08/Chapter-19-Leading-Change-Leadership-Organization-and-Social-Movements.pdf.
28. Available at: https://armstronginstitute.blogs.hopkinsmedicine.org/2013/03/25/a-roadmap-for-patient-safety-and-quality-improvement/.
29. Berwick DM. 100,000 Lives campaign. 2004.
30. Available at: https://www.aci.health.nsw.gov.au/__data/assets/pdf_file/0003/253164/Overview-What_are_PROMs_and_PREMs.pdf.
31. Available at: http://china-ccqc.com/upload/2015-03-12/33fa8a71-12f9-4608-a002-47356efc890f.pdf.

Diffusing Innovation and Best Practice in Health Care

Philip E. Greilich, MD[a],*, Mary Eleanor Phelps, MA, RN[b], William Daniel, MD[c]

KEYWORDS

- Health care • Diffusion • Spreading • Scaling • Quality improvement • Patient safety
- Implementation

KEY POINTS

- All too often, successful quality improvement (QI) pilot projects fail to be diffused or "spread" throughout the system.
- The inability to diffuse successful pilot projects wastes valuable resources, discourages teams and undermines an organization's ability to reduce preventable harms.
- The necessary and sufficient conditions for diffusion require executive leadership, a conducive culture, and the capacity for robust QI.
- Successful diffusion of best practices generally deploys a series of key components over 2-3 major phases.
- Leaders in perioperative medicine will need to adapt the best practice approaches covered in this chapter to help secure the vitality of their organizations during this period of rapid transformation.

INTRODUCTION

Health care systems have extensive portfolios of quality improvement (QI) projects at various stages of execution. Within perioperative medicine, these projects are aimed at reducing errors, infections, transfusions; improving care transfers; enhancing recovery after surgery; and improving outcomes and financial performance. Considerable excitement is generated when pilot projects achieve their stated goals, meet or surpass targets, and finish on time within the defined budget. All too often, however,

Disclosure Statement: None of the authors have a relationship with a commercial company that has direct financial interest in subject matter or materials discussed in the article or with a company making a competing product.

[a] Department of Anesthesiology and Pain Management, University of Texas Southwestern Medical Center, 5323 Harry Hines Boulevard, Dallas, TX 75390, USA; [b] Office of the Associate Dean for Quality, Safety, and Outcomes Education, University of Texas Southwestern Medical Center, 5323 Harry Hines Boulevard, Dallas, TX 75390, USA; [c] Office of the Executive Vice President for Health System Affairs, University of Texas Southwestern Medical Center, 5323 Harry Hines Boulevard, Dallas, TX 75390, USA
* Corresponding author.
E-mail address: Philip.Greilich@UTSouthwestern.edu

Anesthesiology Clin 36 (2018) 127–141
https://doi.org/10.1016/j.anclin.2017.10.009
1932-2275/18/© 2017 Elsevier Inc. All rights reserved.

anesthesiology.theclinics.com

project leaders and teams become frustrated when successful local improvements and best practices are not used by other units within the same department or hospital. As a result, project teams can feel deflated and the failure to spread successful initiatives represents a significant opportunity loss for the organization. Over the past decade, many project teams across health systems in the United States have suffered similar fates despite the documentation of an increasing number of small-scale successes. The inability to scale up or diffuse best practices might explain why medical errors continue to produce substantial morbidity, pain, and distress 15 years after the Institute of Medicine's call to action.[1–6]

Projects are temporary endeavors with a defined beginning and an end. Project teams are often tasked with complex projects that encompass multiple elements and stakeholders. Many health care providers are members of QI project teams and are well-equipped to plan, execute, and complete a QI project. Why then do these fail to spread or be sustained? Often, scaling up and spreading the improvements are not considered in the scope of the project. During project closeout, project teams transfer ownership of the project to process owners within operational units or functional departments. Without additional planning and institutional support, or if teams neglect to define where the responsibility for spreading rests, improvements are at risk of not scaling up, not spreading, and regressing back to the former state. Reverting to ineffective processes or work environments is a waste of resources and may even increase the resistance to subsequent initiatives to improve care. Institutional memory is not sufficient to sustain or spread improvements. Managing spread is an active process requiring careful planning, preparation, and institutional support.

Diffusion is the scientific term for spread and historically has been studied as passive or unmanaged diffusion. Diffusion must be actively managed to be successful in health care.[7,8] Few health care providers have the leverage to make global changes to disseminate best practices across an organization. The propagation of innovation and best practices must help organizations achieve specific goals, so it is essential to articulate the business case showing how the particular best practice makes sense at multiple levels and to different stakeholders. The potential impact of managed diffusion within health care is beginning to emerge. Building the framework for its application in perioperative medicine is the focus of this article.

Active diffusion invokes systems thinking within an organization. It takes into account the dynamic interactions between people, the environment, processes, and outcomes. The factors that shape the context in which the practice is planted also influence the successful diffusion of the practice. Diffusion within a complex sociotechnical system also requires leadership and cultural transformation. Essential drivers of managed diffusion include executive-level engagement, robust QI, operational implementation, monitoring and reporting of outcomes, and knowledge management.[9–12] Knowledge management is a relatively new concept that focuses on the process of acquiring, creating, and sharing knowledge within an organization to achieve its objectives.[13] Diffusion is further enabled when frontline providers are actively engaged, healthy social systems nurtured, and learning readily shared.

This article describes a systematic approach to diffusion within perioperative medicine. It synthesizes work done by the Baldrige Foundation, the Institute for Healthcare Improvement, The Joint Commission Center for Transforming Healthcare, implementation scientists, and health care systems with robust QI programs.[9–16] A case study is used to illustrate the significant phases and critical components of an effective strategy for actively managing diffusion of best practices in a perioperative setting.

ASSESSMENT OF READINESS FOR DIFFUSION

Health care organizations vary widely in their journey toward continuous QI. Ballard[17] describes 4 stages of organization maturity for QI: initiation, foundation building, operationalizing, and continuous QI. Leadership, culture, and infrastructure development represent some of the critical components of this matrix. The first step in preparing for diffusion is to assess an organization's level of maturity because this will have the greatest impact on its capacity for diffusing best practices. A characteristic of mature organizations is the capacity to manage diffusion, which does not generally begin until the organization reaches at least the operationalizing stage of organizational maturity.

The Baldrige framework for quality and performance excellence and The Joint Commission Center for Transforming Health program for high reliability[17,18] place great emphasis on the central role health care executives and senior leaders must play in fostering the learning environment required to achieve high reliability. This includes cultivating a transformative culture and building an infrastructure capable of facilitating the diffusion of knowledge and innovation within the organization. Perioperative leaders need to establish a clear understanding of the style, philosophy, model, and the executive sponsor's commitment to continuous improvement before establishing the scope of a spread project. Fully engaged executive sponsors can be particularly helpful for larger projects when uninformed optimism or pseudo-commitment by senior leaders gives way to the inevitable conflict associated with any significant change process.

Culture is a powerful tool for consistency, but it can be a barrier when innovation is needed to meet new challenges. An institution's culture of safety can be assessed using a validated survey instrument. The most widely used survey is designed and administered by the Agency for Healthcare Research and Quality (AHRQ) every 2 years.[19] This survey measures responses to 42 items in 12 areas that are composites of patient safety issues, medical errors, and event reporting. The toolkit accompanying this survey assists with prioritizing and creating action plans based on survey results. Several of these composites can be used to assess the conditions necessary for spread. These include "management support for patient safety," "supervisor/manager expectations and actions promoting patient safety," "teamwork within units" and "team across units". For diffusion to thrive, these measures need to either be high or showing an improving trend. It is worth noting that improving measures of culture are the result of adapting, adopting, and disseminating team-based tasks. This sounds like a catch-22 (between culture and successful change), yet focuses the "starting point" (and analysis) on what it takes to execute recurring tasks reliably. Processes, priorities, and culture are a response to what it takes to achieve this end, rather than the cause of the change.[20,21]

The infrastructure required for diffusion will vary based on the scope of the project and complexity of the organization. Within perioperative medicine, diffusion of best practices usually involves multiple medical specialties across several clinical and business units. As such, the infrastructure requirements are much more sophisticated than those required for smaller projects. In addition to executive sponsors and project managers, diffusion teams need experienced physician leaders with dedicated time for this work. These physicians frequently work in small groups with nurses and/or administrators with operational experience or assigned responsibility to the involved units. In many cases, subject matter experts in QI, systems engineering, education, information technology, data analytics, and human factors are also required based on the scope and complexity of the project. Clear expectations and budgeted time for clinical staff are essential. Exposing as much of the workforce as possible to basic quality improvement education helps to recruit innovators, early adopters, and champions for the project, as well as provides the workforce needed to drive diffusion.

A stakeholder analysis using a structured set of questions is the second major factor in assessing readiness for diffusion.[18,22] Stakeholders, whose influence on the workforce and environment need to be considered, include department chairs, medical and nursing leaders, division directors, service line executives, QI and patient safety officers, nursing governance council members, and standing QI committee members. Face-to-face interviews may facilitate spread efforts in large departments of anesthesiology and perioperative service lines. **Table 1** provides a series of structured questions that can be used to assess the necessary conditions for spread.

DIFFUSION BEST PRACTICE CASE STUDY

Perioperative care transfers (handoffs or handovers) are a national patient safety priority. Most anesthesiology departments and practices are considering or actively working on improving handoffs to reduce information loss, delays in diagnosis or treatment, and poor teamwork. As successful pilots are completed, a strategy for getting ready for, developing, executing, and refining a diffusion strategy will need to follow. In this case study, an initial effort to diffuse or spread perioperative handoffs in multiple locations is described. Although considerable effort went into preparing and planning this project, execution took much longer than anticipated and encountered significant

Table 1	
Assessing readiness for diffusion: necessary and sufficient conditions for success	
Leadership	• Project activities are identified and aligned with an organizational strategic imperative • Project performance expectations, review criteria, and incentives are in place • Infrastructure with authority to standardize the practice using collective and authority-based decision making
Culture	• Adopters share the understanding that new problems will be appropriately addressed through disseminating innovation and best practices • Clinical best practices are understood by adopters • Process is in place for debriefing and sharing of successes and failures of successful pilot projects
Systems Engineering	• Capability to assess workflow, human factors and usability, technology, outcomes, impact, process engineering and to perform workload modeling • Process for managing implementation; experience and process for actively managing diffusion
Human resources	• Protected time is budgeted for spread project leaders and managers, clinician leads and other support (subject matter experts, administrative assistants, and others). • Access to subject matter experts (QI, education, system engineering, human factors, marketing, information technology) in place
Information Technology	• Decision support that prompts essential information within workflow
Data Analytics	• Access to defined patient, provider, and organizational outcomes • Plan for tracking completeness and coverage of planned spread
Health Service Research	• Ability to analyze if care innovation or best practice indeed improved care or sub-optimized another process

challenges as it transitioned from the pilot site to its first diffusion location. The critical components for diffusion best practices, summarized in **Table 2**, will serve as a template for the case study and the debriefing that follows. The elements in the table represent a summary of the framework for spread endorsed by the Institute for Healthcare Improvement (IHI) and the Model for Diffusion used successfully by the Mayo Clinic for value creation.[9,10,15,16,23]

Table 2 Framework for managed diffusion		
Phase	**Key Component**	**Activity**
Getting Ready	*Leadership*	*Identify project's alignment with institution's strategic plan*
	1. Alignment	• Recruit an executive sponsor who is accountable for delivering this organizational strategic objective
	2. Executive Sponsor	• Designate a day-to-day spread leader
	3. Day-to-day manager teams	• Create steering team and spread teams with a mix of expertise and secure the funding required to support the spread project
Developing Spread Plan	*Organizational set-up*	*Carefully select and support pilot unit to ensure their goals are successfully achieved*
	1. Success ideas	• Description of what is being spread (processes, innovations)
	2. Aim statement	• Target unit(s), timeframe, target level of performance
	3. Assess readiness	• Assess organizational readiness and risk of implementation, complexity of intervention
	4. Detailed plan	• Full scale in mind, impact of centralized vs. consensus approach on timeline, kickoff timetable, leverage of pilot units on spread units, recruitment of formal and informal leaders, infrastructure enhancements (EMR, cognitive aids), tracking of completeness and coverage, linkage to operational bodies during/after rollout
	Communication	*Develop a communication plan*
	1. Audience/channels	• Identify all the target audiences and communication channels (meetings, displays, electronic) to attract adopters
	2. Leaders/units	• Set-up opportunities for leaders to communicate with target units and for target unit to communicate with leaders
	3. Justify expectations	• Provide information to support action/set clear expectations
	Nurturing social system	*Recruit unit-based champions, influencers, mentors and willing volunteers from each significant stakeholder group and makes plans to engage using preferred communication style*
	Measurement	*Changes in system performance: metrics/ display linked to aims and extent/rate of spread*

(continued on next page)

Phase	Key Component	Activity
Table 2 **(*continued*)**		
Executing and Refining the Spread Plan	*Feedback*	*Regular collection of data and activities on unit and feedback to and from frontline providers; validate subsets of automated reports to ensure accuracy*
	1. Reporting	• Sharing summary reports (dashboards) with executive sponsor, senior leaders and across organization (intranet) at pre-existing reporting forums (meetings, reports)
	2. Adjust as needed	• Progress slower/faster than expected; determine cause (education, measurement system, vitality of pilot unit, creation/movement of new ideas) to guide adjustment
	3. Sustain the gains	• Hold senior leadership responsible; maintain alignment with strategic goals by regular review of dashboard(s) linked to organizational balanced scorecard • Revise policy/procedures and imbed QI activity into operations and provide performance incentives to ensure corrective actions occur with ongoing feedback

Abbreviation: EMR, electronic medical record.
Data from Refs.[9,10,15,16,23]

Case Study: Leadership

This project was initially selected as a clinical practicum for an institutionally sponsored clinical safety and effectiveness course. The project leader and nursing unit manager attended a 6-month, in-house session and learned basic quality improvement skills to help recruit a team and complete the project. Topic selection was voluntary and, in this case, handoffs from the cardiovascular operating room (OR) to cardiovascular intensive care unit (ICU) were chosen because the course participants worked in these units and handoffs had been identified as a latent safety threat. The initial cycle of improvement spanned 6 months. Provider satisfaction scores indicated that having a more structured handoff process and checklist addressed a significant gap in care coordination. Adoption, however, was incomplete. Attitudes and behaviors varied significantly among providers. In response, a second, more comprehensive cycle of improvement was designed that included plans for spreading the process, tasks, and behaviors throughout the department of anesthesiology and perioperative service line. The physician leader from the initial cycle remained with the project and an experienced research coordinator was added to the team. A department chair was recruited as the executive sponsor. Letters of support were written by division directors, other chairmen, the chief nursing officer, and the hospital chief quality officer. A proposal for extramural funding was submitted from the statewide health care system. These funds provided partial support for a project coordinator and nonclinical time for physician and nursing leads. A steering (design) team composed of subject matter experts with backgrounds in education, team training, human factors, and medical informatics was assembled to guide diffusion teams from each clinical location. Volunteers for a multispecialty diffusion team were recruited from anesthesiology, critical care medicine, nursing, and surgery, which included nurses and doctors with a wide range of experience, to redesign the handoff process at the pilot and initial diffusion site.

Organizational Set-Up

The cardiovascular OR and ICU units were again selected as the pilot unit given the successful initial cycle of improvement. A series of concurrent QI activities designed to promote teamwork and patient safety were also planned as part of a national collaborative. This unit had a history of involving medical students, residents, and faculty in QI projects to fulfill medical education and promotion requirements. New ideas included the use of participatory ergonomics in the form of steering [design] team used to guide the diffusion teams; systems engineering to improve patients safety (SEIPS); multimodal, multidimensional education and training; cognitive aids; and information technology (ie, our medical record [EMR]).[24,25] The project charter outlined the formation of a departmental collaborative to spread perioperative handoff redesign to four adult inpatient hospitals affiliated with the health system. The stated aim was to reduce harms attributed to handoffs. The initial performance measure was to minimize information loss during handoffs by 50% in 2 ICUs in 2 hospitals in 18 months. A series of introductory presentations were made to all involved units, departments, and stakeholders. A detailed plan timeline (Gantt chart) for the redesign and spread process was formulated. The strategy was to use multispecialty teams (consensus approach) to customize the essential components of a structured handoff process for their respective units and recruit their peers to assist with change management.

Communication

A weekly face-to-face meeting between the project leader and coordinator and bimonthly teleconference with the diffusion team served as the primary means of communication, action planning, feedback, and follow-up. Attendance varied, so minutes were distributed bimonthly to every member of the departmental collaborative. Executive leadership did not attend group meetings but were provided updates approximately every 6 months. A presentation made to the surgical services executive committee (department chairs) was met with skepticism by some influential members of this group. Flyers were used periodically to announce projects events. The project was branded as enhanced communication for handoffs from the OR to the ICU (ECHO-ICU).

Nurturing Social Systems

Multispecialty representation on the diffusion teams facilitated recruitment of peers to serve as champions. A series of multidisciplinary team training exercises were used to promote a learning environment and serve as a means testing usability and identifying failure modes.

Measurement, Feedback, and Knowledge Management

The charter outlined a panel of process, provider, patient, and organizational outcomes. Support for data management and analysis was made possible by extramural funding. Video recording of handoffs, use of distinct evaluation forms, and an observer training process permitted asynchronous grading of conformance to the new process. The project team collected qualitative and quantitative feedback from bedside providers on an annual basis. Standardized education material was constructed for use on Web-based training encompassing onboarding, yearly training and multilevel education for students, trainees. Unit-based policies and procedures were revised to reflect the redesigned handoff process. Lesson learned were shared during the bimonthly meetings. A protected share drive housed all the support material needed for redesign and implementation.

Debriefing: Getting Ready

The chief shortcoming of the initial phase of the project was not identifying the alignment between perioperative care transfers and a key strategic imperative within the organization, such as an organization-wide campaign to close gaps in care coordination or to build a culture of high reliability. Given the scope of the project, its executive sponsor needed a high-priority internal lever to mobilize the resources and political will required. Letters of recommendation are fine but may not be sufficient to sway senior leaders who suffer from a constant barrage of requests for financial assistance and political coverage. The ideal condition would be to have an executive owner of an aligned organizational imperative as the project sponsor. This directly aligns the strategic priority with access to the needed resources. An executive sponsor who is also a senior executive within the organization would be in a better position to moderate resistance from operational leadership when dialogue is required to address skepticism or conflict. Finally, active involvement and visible presence of an executive sponsor provides first-hand knowledge of the importance of the project and serves as an opportunity to mentor future leaders on early detection and management of risk and reward.

Developing Spread Plan

The ideas, aim statement, charter, and detailed plan all looked good on paper and were validated by receipt of external funding for the project. A comprehensive assessment of readiness and performance of a failure modes analysis would have provided project leaders a more realistic, understanding of the environmental conditions and given them an opportunity to anticipate and plan for potential resistance.[26] With this knowledge, the scope and complexity of the project may have been revised. That is to say, modify the scope to cover intraoperative instead of interdepartmental handoffs, or simulation training only versus full implementation.

Communication with all relevant stakeholders, especially senior leadership was insufficient given the scope of the project. Periodic review of the project with senior leaders, using spread trackers (see **Fig. 1**) and status reports, could have been use to inform them better and elicit their guidance and support. Equally important, the provision of "talking points" during these sessions would have armed them with information needed to manage resistors, especially other senior leaders better. For the frontline staff, multi-modal communication using display boards, online videos, such as YouTube, and newsletters were needed to supplement the use of more traditional approaches such as email communications and face-to-face meetings given their limitations.

Tracking and measuring the speed and extent of spread is equally as important as measuring more traditional outcomes (process, providers, patients, organizational). In this case, it may have prompted an earlier reassessment and adjustment. The use of a spread tracker, shown in **Fig. 1**, is a best practice that allows demonstration of completeness and coverage of a spread effort.[10]

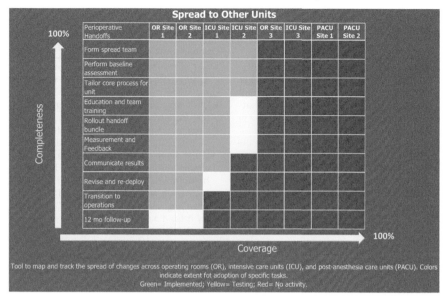

Fig. 1. Spread tracker used to show coverage and completeness across several clinical areas. (*Adapted from* Schall MW, Chappell C, Nielsen GA, et al. Transforming care at the bedside how-to-guide: Spreading innovations to improve care on medical and surgical units. Cambridge (MA): Institute for Healthcare Improvement; 2008. Available at: http://www.ihi.org/resources/Pages/Tools/TCABHowToGuideSpreadingInnovations.aspx. Accessed October 30, 2017; with permission.)

Debriefing: Executing and Refining the Spread Plan

This project remains at high risk for experiencing a short half-life if operational ownership and adoption do not occur. A stable reporting system such as dashboard or diffusion tracker needs to be constructed and reviewed on a regular basis in regularly scheduled reporting forums (reports, meetings). The steering team also needs to maintain the bandwidth to promote adjustments and to preserve the vitality of the pilot unit(s) to ensure the pace and momentum of the diffusion teams. Completeness and coverage of the intended diffusion are unlikely to occur unless the executive sponsor and senior leadership can align this effort with an organizational strategic imperative. Additional tips for completeness and coverage are summarized in **Table 3**. Periodic measurement of conformance with the new handover process could be achieved by designing observer-training program for trainees, staff, and physicians interested in fulfilling QI requirements within their curriculum or for promotion, recertification, and recredentialing.

DEVELOPING CAPACITY FOR DIFFUSION (SPREAD)

Most health care institutions have yet to build the capacity for diffusing innovation and best practices within their organizations. Those actively involved in doing so are working to pool external resources and restructure the use of human resources and organizational operations to meet this growing demand. Much of the evidence on how to diffuse best practice in health care is just beginning to emerge. Some of these early explorations include improvements in organizational ergonomics, participation in peer-to-peer learning collaboratives, and examination of diffusion team composition and executive-level skills needed to lead sociotechnical change in complex systems.

Table 3	
Elements to consider for coverage and completeness	
Coverage	**Completeness**
• Keep executive leadership engaged with spread tracker and bulleted talking points. • Constancy of purpose: set the expectation that leadership will keep asking and that staff cannot wait out this special project or flavor of the month. • Be mindful of change fatigue and pace the rollout. • Build in necessary redundancies in the system to catch lapses in spread. • Create a visual display of coverage and completeness to track progress.	• Get the vital few on board (most will follow). The remainder will need to be managed. • Understand what prevents the remaining few from coming on board. • Use your champions and quickly find a success story. Measure and spread the word. Some of the most effective champions are the ones who are former holdouts. • Start small with the skeptical and unwilling, asking questions like "Will you try it for a day?" • Use leadership to force the issue. Be straightforward and ask, 　"Do you know something that we do not? If you do, we need to understand it. If not, you need to get on board."

Examples of external resources include publications on diffusion projects and participation in peer-to-peer learning collaboratives.[23,27–30] Given its formative stage, diffusion in health care will likely require experimentation between innovators and spreaders.[31,32] Some early examples of these efforts are starting to appear in the literature. Other resources are emerging, such as web-based invitations to participate in multicenter learning collaboratives. **Table 4** summarizes some of the resources relevant to perioperative medicine. Participation in a learning collaborative is a particularly attractive option because it provides an immersive experiencing diffusion projects supported by national experts and provides access to lessons learned from other institutions undergoing similar exercises. It can also be very helpful in gaining local support for diffusion project by leveraging the reputations of and even possibly engaging competition among participating centers.

Organizational ergonomics plays a central role in applying a systems approach to build capacity for diffusing innovation and best practices. The use of participatory ergonomics to guide spread teams, pathways for channeling human resources within a service line to meet institutional priorities, and restructuring operations to support care across multiple medical specialties and clinical units all serve to improve organizational ergonomics. Participatory ergonomics is an organizational macroergonomic that uses steering (design) teams, functioning at a departmental, service-line, or health system level, to guide unit-based spread teams in the diffusion of important best practices. This model has been used efficiently on the regional and national scale by the AHRQ (Michigan Keystone ICU project)[39] and the IHI (5 Million Lives Campaign).[44] More recently, the American Society of Anesthesiology has launched a similar effort to support the development of the perioperative surgical home.[27] The most successful regional application was the Keystone ICU project that promoted a series of interventions that included daily rounds, a comprehensive unit-based safety team program, and central line and ventilator bundles) to encourage teamwork and reduce morbidity in more than 108 ICUs in 77 hospitals in the state of Michigan.[39–41] Xie and colleagues[24] recently demonstrated the use of participatory ergonomics to spread the use of family-centered rounds within a hospital.

Table 4
Literature and Web-based resources

Topic	Available Material	Reference
Spread framework Diffusion model	IHI Framework for Spread Consolidated Framework for Implementation Research Mayo Clinic Value Creation Baylor Healthcare Care System Journey	Roger 1995,[6] Schall 2008[8] Million Hearts Campaign[29] Damschroeder 2009[9] Swensen 2009,[14] Swensen 2012[13] Ballard 2014[17]
Safe surgery checklists	State-wide spread project in 14 South Carolina inpatient hospitals	Haynes 2017,[33] Molina 2016[34]
Enhanced recovery after surgery (ERAS)	Spread project aims to help hospital adopt ERAS using comprehensive unit-based safety program (CUSP) method	Ahrq.gov/professionals/quality-patient-safety/hais/tools/enhanced-recovery/index.html[35]
Care transfer handoffs, handovers	TJC, Center for Transforming Care Toolkit Large-scale implementation of IPASS	TST 2015,[28] Benjamin 2016[36] Shahian 2017,[37] Starmer 2014[38]
Hospital-associated infections (HAIs)	Spread project to reduce HAIs in 108 ICUs in 77 hospitals in Michigan Keystone Project	Pronovost 2006,[39] AHRQ CUSP[29] Goeschel 2008,[40] Berenholtz 2011[41]
Patient blood management (PBM)	Spread of PBM in a health care system PBM implementation strategy	Frank 2017[42] Meybolm 2016[43]

Abbreviations: TJC, The Joint Commission; IPASS, Illness severity, Patient summary, Action list, Situation awareness and contingency planning, Synthesis by receiver.

The composition and capabilities of a diffusion team differ from those of a project team. In a Lean Six Sigma model, a unit-based pilot project would require green-belt level skills for the project lead (physician or nurse) and possibly for the project champion and process owner. Diffusion projects in complex health care systems, however, are likely to benefit from Six Sigma black-belt level project manager and subject matter experts in systems engineering, multidisciplinary education and training, data analytics, QI, patient safety, and human factors. In academic medical centers, health services research specialists should be included to bring scientific rigor to the project. The goals should be to create a reproducible methodology and processes with results capable of influencing teams both internally and externally.

The systematic diffusion of best practices across a large department, practice, or service line requires executive-level leadership skills. This work demands strategic alignment, planning, and organizational authority to help control conflict and provide direction and protection for those executing this work. This frequently requires the ability to formulate proposals, business plan, that includes demonstrable returns on investment. This work also needs an enterprise-level lens. The benefits of a spread project must be weighed against its impact on other important financial, patient satisfaction, staff engagement, or patient safety measures. If funded, spread projects within the perioperative service will likely require spread leaders to reach across multiple specialties, clinical, and business units within the perioperative service line. To meet this need, Pronovost and colleagues[45] argue that a new tier of physician leadership must be created to perform the executive functions required for complex activities, like active diffusion. The demands of transforming health care in complex organizations will likely require roles such as a vice chair for patient safety and QI for large departments or an associate medical director for patient safety and QI for service lines. This individual will play a vital role in promoting the bidirectional communication and coordination needed between health system chief quality officers, medical school (vice, associate) deans (for QI education), and operational leadership.

LIMITATIONS AND FUTURE RESEARCH

The evidence base on technical (content) and adaptive (contextual) factors for successful diffusion and is limited but emerging.[46,47] Although implementation scientists have constructed a model for its study (CFIR), its application in the perioperative setting has not been tested.[11] Given this, future research will need to focus on investigating the effectiveness of interventions promoting diffusion, focuses on the evaluation of contextual factors, leverages the electronic medical record data and tools, and uses of qualitative and observational methodologies is needed.[46] By necessity, this work requires a shift away from traditional randomized controlled trials towards those with more pragmatic, qualitative and observational designs. This will provide us with a better understanding of the contextual factors and other drivers that influence successful diffusion of best practice.[46,48] This will necessitate the measurement of organizational or practice context; the involvement of stakeholders and leadership; implementation of scope, duration, timing; and the completeness and coverage of diffusion on outcomes. Interested readers are encouraged to learn more about the journal *Implementation Science* and consider attending the Annual Conference on the Science of Dissemination and Implementation in Health (cohosted by AcademyHealth and the National Institutes of Health) to explore a partnership with those seeking clinical sites.

SUMMARY

Timely and efficient diffusion of innovation and best practice within perioperative medicine is one of the most demanding and elusive aspect of realizing the full potential of a successful pilot project. It is best to start with an assessment of organizational readiness to determine if the necessary and sufficient conditions for diffusion are present for a given project. Recommendations from the Baldrige Foundation, the IHI, and The Joint Commission, implementation science and health care systems with robust QI programs provide guidance on how these principles can be applied to the perioperative setting. Active management of diffusion within a large private practice organizations, academic departments, and service lines requires careful preparation, planning, execution, and refining by skilled managers and executive leadership. There are several opportunities to build an organization's capacity for diffusion or spread if it is willing to invest in the training and undergo some restructuring to support this essential activities. Perioperative leaders are encouraged to look for opportunities to accelerate their growth by participating in learning collaboratives designed to spread best practices such as safe surgery, enhanced recovery after surgery, handoffs, and comprehensive unit-based safety team programs. The ability to rapidly and efficiently scale up a successful pilot could dramatically increase the impact of our work and allow us to measure our success in lives saved.

ACKNOWLEDGMENTS

The authors would like to thank Gary Reed, MD, Charles Whitten, MD, John McCracken, PhD, Paul Convery, MD and Michael Deegan, MD for their review and guidance with this work and article.

REFERENCES

1. Makary MA, Daniel M. Medical error—the third leading cause of death in the US. BMJ 2016;353:i2139.
2. James JT. A new, evidence-based estimate of patient harms associated with hospital care. J Patient Saf 2013;9(3):122–8.
3. Classen DC, Resar R, Griffin F, et al. 'Global trigger tool' shows that adverse events in hospitals may be ten times greater than previously measured. Health Aff 2011;30(4):581–9.
4. Long SJ, Brown KF, Ames D, et al. What is known about adverse events in older medical hospital inpatients? A systematic review of the literature. Int J Qual Health Care 2013;25(5):542–54.
5. Bergman LM, Pettersson ME, Chaboyer WP, et al. Safety hazards during intrahospital transport: a prospective observational study. Crit Care Med 2017;45(10): e1043–9.
6. Institute of Medicine Committee on Quality of Health Care in A. In: Crossing the Quality Chasm: A New Health System for the 21st Century. Washington (DC): National Academies Press (US) Copyright 2001 by the National Academy of Sciences. All rights reserved. 2001.
7. Rogers E. Diffusion of innovations. 4th edition. New York: The Free Press; 1995.
8. Greenhalgh T, Robert G, Macfarlane F, et al. Diffusion of innovations in service organizations: systematic review and recommendations. Milbank Q 2004;82: 581–629.
9. Massoud MR, Nielsen GA, Nolan K, et al. A framework for spread: from local improvements to system-wide change. IHI innovation series white paper. Cambridge (MA): Institute for Healthcare Improvement; 2006. Available at: http://www.IHI.org/IHI/Results/WhitePapers/AFrameworkforSpreadWhitePaper.htm.
10. Schall MW, Chappell C, Nielsen GA, et al. Transforming care at the bedside how-to-guide: spreading innovations to improve care on medical and surgical units. Cambridge(MA): Institute for Healthcare Improvement; 2008. Available at: http://www.IHI.org.
11. Damschroder LJ, Aron DC, Keith RE, et al. Fostering implementation of health services research findings into practice: a consolidated framework for advancing implementation science. Implement Sci 2009;4:50.
12. Baldrige Performance Excellence Program. 2017-2018 Baldrige Excellence Framework (Health Care). Available at: https://www.nist.gov/baldrige/publications/baldrige-excellence-framework/health-care.
13. Knowledge management. Available at: http://www.unc.edu/~sunnyliu/inls258/Introduction_to_Knowledge_Management.html; https://web.archive.org/web/20070319233812/.
14. Nolan K, Schall M, Erb F, et al. Using a framework for spread: the case of patient access in the Veterans Health Administration. Jt Comm J Qual Patient Saf 2005; 31:339–47. Available at: www.jcrinc.com.
15. Swensen SJ, Dilling JA, Harper CM, et al. The Mayo Clinic value system creation system. Am J Med Qual 2012;27:58–65.
16. Swensen SJ, Dilling JA, Milliner DS, et al. Quality: the Mayo approach. Am J Med Qual 2009;24:428–40.
17. Ballard. Achieving STEEEP Health Care. New York: Productivity Press; 2013.
18. Oro™ 2.0 High Reliability Assessment and Resources. Joint Commission Center for Transforming Healthcare. Available at: https://www.nist.gov/baldrige/publications/baldrige-excellence-framework/health-care.

19. HSOPS Hospital Survey on Patient Safety Culture. Agency for Healthcare Research and Quality. Available at: https://www.ahrq.gov/professionals/quality-patient-safety/patientsafetyculture/hospital/index.html.

20. Christensen, Clayton M, Shu K. What Is an Organization's Culture? Harvard Business School Background Note 399-104, February 1999. (Revised August 2006).

21. Schein E. Organizational culture and leadership. San Francisco: Jossey-Bass Publishers; 1988. Chapters 1–3.

22. Rutherford P, Phillips J, Coughlan P, et al. Transforming care at the bedside how-to guide: engaging front-line staff in innovation and quality improvement. Cambridge (MA): Institute for Healthcare Improvement; 2008. Available at: http://www.ihi.org/Topics/MedicalSurgicalCare/MedicalSurgicalCareGeneral/Tools/TCABHowToGuideEngagingStaff.htm.

23. IHI Spreading improvements in health care. Available at: http://www.ihi.org/Topics/Spread/Pages/default.aspx.

24. Xie A, Carayon P, Cox ED, et al. Application of participatory ergonomics to the redesign of the family-centered rounds process. Ergonomics 2015;58:1726–44.

25. Holden RJ, Carayon P, Gurses AP, et al. SEIPS 2.0: a human factors framework for studying and improving the work of healthcare professionals and patients. Ergonomics 2013;56(11):1669–86.

26. Freitag M, Carroll VS. Handoff communication: using failure modes and effects analysis to improve the transition in care process. Qual Manag Health Care 2011;20:10309.

27. American Society of Anesthesiology. Perioperative Surgical Home Learning Collaborative. Available at: https://www.asahq.org/psh/learning%20collaborative.

28. Targeted Solutions Tool® for Handoff Communications. Joint Commission Center for Transforming Healthcare. 2015. Available at: http://www.centerfortransforminghealthcare.org/tst_hoc.aspx.

29. Agency for Healthcare Research and Quality. Comprehensive Unit-Based Safety Program (CUSP) Toolkit. Available at: https://www.ahrq.gov/professionals/education/curriculum-tools/cusptoolkit/index.html.

30. Running a Successful Campaign in Your Hospital. How-to-Guide. 100,000 Lives Campaign. Institute for Healthcare Improvement. Available at: http://www.ihi.org/IHI/Programs/Campaign/.

31. Connect innovators with spreaders. AHRQ Health Care Innovations Exchange. Available at: https://innovations.ahrq.gov/MillionHeartsReport/report2.

32. Millions Hearts Campaign™: Scaling and spreading innovation: Strategies to improve cardiovascular health. Available at: https://innovations.ahrq.gov/scale-up-and-spread/reports/scaling-and-spreading-innovation-strategies-improve-cardiovascular.

33. Haynes AB, Edmondson L, Lipsitz SR, et al. Mortality trends after a voluntary checklist-based surgical safety collaborative. Ann Surg 2017. https://doi.org/10.1097/SLA.0000000000002249.

34. Molina G, Jiang W, Edmondson L, et al. Implementation of the surgical surgery checklist in South Carolinas is associated with improvement in perceived patient safety. J Am Coll Surg 2016;222:725–36.

35. AHRQ Safety Program for Improving Surgical Care and Recover: A collaborative program to enhance the recovery of surgical patients. Available at: http://www.Ahrq.gov/professionals/quality-patient-safety/hais/tools/enhanced-recovery/index.html.

36. Benjamin MF, Hargrave S, Nether K. Using the targeted solutions tool to improve emergency department handoffs in a community hospital. Jt Comm J Qual Patient Saf 2016;42:107–14.
37. Shahian DM, McEachern K, Rossi L, et al. Large-scale implementation of the IPASS handover system at an academic medical center. BMJ Qual Saf 2017; 26:760–70.
38. Starmer AJ, Spector ND, Srivastava R, et al. Changes in medical errors after implementation of a handoff program. N Engl J Med 2014;371:1803–12.
39. Pronovost P, Needham D, Berenholtz S, et al. An intervention to decrease catheter-related bloodstream infections in the ICU. N Engl J Med 2006;355: 2725–32.
40. Goeschel CA, Pronovost P. Harnessing the potential of health care collaboratives: lesson from the Keystone ICU project. In: Henriksen K, Battles JB, Keyes MA, et al, editors. Advances in patient safety: new directions and alternative approaches: culture and redesign, vol. 2. Rockville (MD): Agency for Healthcare Research and Quality; 2008.
41. Berenholtz SM, Pham JC, Thompson DA, et al. Collaborative Cohort Study of an Intervention to Reduce Ventilator-Associated Pneumonia in the Intensive Care Unit. Infect Control Hosp Epidemiol 2011;32:305–14.
42. Frank S, Thakkar RN, Podlasek SJ, et al. Implementing a health system-wide patient blood management program with a clinical community approach. Anesthesiology 2017. https://doi.org/10.1097/ALN.0000000000001851.
43. Meybolm P, Richards T, Isbister J, et al. Patient blood management bundles to facilitate implementation. Transfus Med Rev 2017;31:62–71.
44. Million Lives Campaign. Institutes for Healthcare Improvement. Available at: http://www.ihi.org/Engage/Initiatives/Completed/5MillionLivesCampaign/Pages/default.aspx.
45. Pronovost P, Miller M, Wachter RM, et al. Perspective: physician leadership in quality. Acad Med 2009;84:1651–6.
46. Kaplan HC, Brady PW, Dritz MC, et al. The influence of context on quality improvement success in health care: a systematic review of the literature. Milbank Q 2010;88:500–59.
47. Chan WV, Pearson TA, Bennett GC, et al. ACC/AHA Special Report: Clinical practice guideline implementation strategies: A summary of systematic reviews by the NHLBI implementation science work group. Circulation 2017;135. https://doi.org/10.1161/CIR.0000000000000481.
48. Caruso D, Kerrigan CL, Mastanduno MP, et al. Improving value-based care and outcomes of clinical populations in an electronic health record system environment. A technical report. The Dartmouth Institute for Health Policy and Clinical Practice: 2011.

Moving?

Make sure your subscription moves with you!

To notify us of your new address, find your **Clinics Account Number** (located on your mailing label above your name), and contact customer service at:

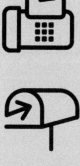

Email: journalscustomerservice-usa@elsevier.com

800-654-2452 (subscribers in the U.S. & Canada)
314-447-8871 (subscribers outside of the U.S. & Canada)

Fax number: 314-447-8029

Elsevier Health Sciences Division
Subscription Customer Service
3251 Riverport Lane
Maryland Heights, MO 63043

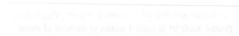

Printed and bound by CPI Group (UK) Ltd, Croydon, CR0 4YY

08/05/2025

01864709-0002